In Clinical Practice

Taking a practical approach to clinical medicine, this series of smaller reference books is designed for the trainee physician, primary care physician, nurse practitioner and other general medical professionals to understand each topic covered. The coverage is comprehensive but concise and is designed to act as a primary reference tool for subjects across the field of medicine.

More information about this series at https://link.springer.com/bookseries/13483

Alberto Martinez-Isla
Lalin Navaratne
Editors

Laparoscopic Common Bile Duct Exploration

Foreword by
Lord Darzi of Denham
Peter B. Cotton

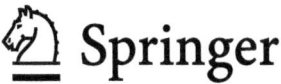 Springer

Editors
Alberto Martinez-Isla
London North West University
Healthcare NHS Trust
London, UK

Lalin Navaratne
London North West University
Healthcare NHS Trust
London, UK

ISSN 2199-6652   ISSN 2199-6660   (electronic)
In Clinical Practice

ISBN 978-3-030-93202-2   ISBN 978-3-030-93203-9   (eBook)
https://doi.org/10.1007/978-3-030-93203-9

This Springer imprint is published by the registered company Springer
Nature Switzerland AG
The registered company address is: Gewerbestrasse 11, 6330 Cham, Switzerland

Foreword by Lord Darzi of Denham

Biliary disease remains one of the most enigmatic areas of human health. The path of bile that originates in the liver and progresses down several anatomical ducts that flow to a variety of structures and organs such as the gallbladder and the small bowel where once considered to be one of the most understood areas of early twentieth century medicine. The system was maintained to be one that released digestive chemicals used in fat absorption and a mechanical blockage in this path would result in an excess of bile that would result in jaundice (icterus).

These diseases have characteristic patterns and associations and can afflict patients through multiple routes affecting the biliary pathway that include bile duct obstruction, autoimmune diseases, hepatitis, and blood disorders in neonates. These are conditions that can affect both genders, all socio-economic classes, all ages, and all nations—an issue that was highlighted at the last *World Innovation Summit for Health* (WISH). In the world of politics, biliary disease has been seen in the United States Presidents Lyndon B. Johnson and James A. Garfield and the prominent British Foreign Secretary Anthony Eden which have been reported as carrying significance on national and international decisions.

In subsequent years, the growth of molecular laboratory techniques, structural biology, enzymology, and metabolism has highlighted the increased complexity of the biliary system. We now understand that bile and its molecular receptors govern a wide variety of cellular metabolic processes whose dysfunction can modulate an extensive range of physiological states that span basal metabolic rate, immune cell activity, gene expression, and multiple hormonal pathways.

Managing biliary disease has therefore grown significantly in the past century, and the birth of minimally invasive approaches that I have personally witnessed and championed (ranging from laparoscopic, endoscopic, and even robotic techniques) has offered whole new paradigms for surgeons to manage biliary obstruction.

During my time as a consultant surgeon, I have seen Alberto Isla innovating in the management of benign obstructive biliary disease. He has done this in an auspicious area of western central London (at St Mary's Hospital at Imperial Healthcare NHS Trust) where, as colleagues, we found ourselves practicing surgery meters away from the site of United Kingdom's first bile duct operation that had historically been performed by John Knowsley Thornton in the nineteenth century.

Alberto has a large surgical experience in biliary operations and has innovated novel techniques to manage obstructive biliary stone disease. These include the LABEL procedure; Lithotripsy-Assisted Bile Duct Exploration by Laparoendoscopy for Choledocholithiasis (where he also first introduced lasers into this part of the anatomy). He has also enhanced transcystic approaches for bile duct exploration.

This book therefore represents the culmination of the author's experience in high volume and advanced bile duct surgery with the laparoscopic approach. It is a wide-ranging text on the origins and evolution of biliary surgery to progressive surgical approaches for managing biliary obstruction. It presents the reader with information to tackle the nuances and complexities of biliary obstruction and gives a vision of where this field is headed in the future. As a practicing surgeon, my early research was in biliary diseases and novel technologies used to manage them. I have continued to be fascinated by this area. I found this book to be a valuable guide to laparoscopic biliary techniques for surgeons, trainees, and those interested in biliary ailments. It represents a platform for continued innovation in biliary surgery and healthcare technology for the foreseeable future and adds to the dissemination of good-quality clinical practice for surgeons faced with biliary disease.

Lord Darzi of Denham, OM PC KBE
FMedSci FREng FRS
Imperial College
London, UK

Foreword by Peter B. Cotton

I have enjoyed reading this scholarly and comprehensive treatise on laparoscopic common bile duct exploration (LCBDE). As a specialist in biliary and pancreatic disorders, I was closely involved in the early discussions and controversies about the optimal treatment strategy for patients with gall bladder stones and suspected choledochal stones. For me, an important question was the role of ERCP, if and when it should be used before, after, or even during cholecystectomy.

The first issue was (and is) how best to define the level of suspicion that stones might be present in the bile duct in patients with choledochlithiasis. Just 30 years ago, using clinical, imaging, and biochemical parameters, we proposed three categories of patients referring to the likelihood of duct stones: i.e. very likely, very unlikely, and intermediate (1,2).

These observations and categories have been argued and refined with numerous research studies, made more intriguing and complex by the availability of MRCP, EUS, and indeed LCBDE (3–7). How patients in the "intermediate" category are treated remains a key practical and controversial question. Is it "best" to do LCBDE or LC + ERCP?

Why still controversial? Surely a large formal randomized trial would provide the answer? However, such a study could only be done by experts in specialist centers, and the results would, therefore, have little relevance to the real world where most surgery is done. Obviously the one-stop LCBDE approach would appear to be ideal, but does not seem to dominate practice, at least in the USA. Chapter 8 in this book highlights the fact that surgery trainees have little exposure to

LCBDE, so that most entering practice are unlikely to embrace it. Many general surgeons prefer to avoid the technical complexity, possible risks, and added OR time, and rely on ERCP post-operatively to remove stones detected by intra-operative cholangiography (8). Whether they are comfortable and right to do so depends very much on the expertise of their local colleagues offering ERCP, which is an issue that has long concerned me.

I have stopped doing procedures now, but my experience of referrals and as an expert in medico-legal cases showed me that not all those doing ERCP were indeed competent. A fundamental problem is that there is no compulsion or indeed mechanism for ERCPists to document and report their performance. A key issue in the USA is that most hospitals do a poor job in credentialing for ERCP, as shown in a recent survey (9).

All this means that patients are at the mercy of practitioners of unknown expertise, and adds relevance to the need for GI surgeons and Gastroenterologists to work closely together, another hobby horse of mine (10). I have been fortunate to have had awesome surgical partners in my career, especially Chris Russell at The Middlesex Hospital in London, Bill Meyers and Ted Pappas at Duke, and David Adams at the Medical University of South Carolina.

As this excellent book shows, LCBDE is an elegant and valuable procedure, but there is an elephant hiding somewhere. In order to expand its use, should cholecystectomy be the purview of pancreatic-biliary surgeons, rather than generalists?

Peter B. Cotton, MD FRCP FRCS
Digestive Disease Center
Medical University of South Carolina
Charleston, SC, USA
http://www.drpetercotton.com

References

1. Cotton PB, Baillie J, Pappas TN, Meyers WS. Laparoscopic cholecystectomy and the biliary endoscopist. Gastrointest Endosc. 1991 Jan-Feb;37(1): 94–7. https://doi.org/10.1016/s0016-5107(91)70637-8. PMID: 1825986.
2. Cotton PB. Endoscopic retrograde cholangiopancreatography and laparoscopic cholecystectomy. Am J Surg. 1993 Apr;165(4):474–8. https://doi.org/10.1016/s0002-9610(05)80944-4. PMID: 8480885.
3. Cotton PB, Chung SC, Davis WZ, Gibson RM, Ransohoff DF, Strasberg SM. Issues in cholecystectomy and management of duct stones. Am J Gastroenterol. 1994 Aug;89(8 Suppl):S169–76. PMID: 8048408.
4. Onken JE, Brazer SR, Eisen GM, Williams DM, Bouras EP, DeLong ER, Long TT 3rd, Pancotto FS, Rhodes DL, Cotton PB. Predicting the presence of choledocholithiasis in patients with symptomatic cholelithiasis. Am J Gastroenterol. 1996 Apr;91(4):762–7. PMID: 8677945.
5. Davis WZ, Cotton PB, Arias R, Williams D, Onken JE. ERCP and sphincterotomy in the context of laparoscopic cholecystectomy: academic and community practice patterns and results. Am J Gastroenterol. 1997 Apr;92(4):597–601. PMID: 9128306.
6. Yu CY, Roth N, Jani N, Cho J, Van Dam J, Selby R, Buxbaum J. Dynamic liver test patterns do not predict bile duct stones. Surg Endosc. 2019 Oct;33(10):3300–313. https://doi.org/10.1007/s00464-018-06620-x. Epub 2019 Mar 25. PMID: 30911921
7. Kadah A, Khoury T, Mahamid M, Assy N, Sbeit W. Predicting common bile duct stones by non-invasive parameters. Hepatobiliary Pancreat Dis Int. 2020 Jun;19(3):266–70. https://doi.org/10.1016/j.hbpd.2019.11.003. Epub 2019 Nov 20. PMID: 31810810.
8. ASGE Standards of Practice Committee, Buxbaum JL, Abbas Fehmi SM, Sultan S, Fishman DS, Qumseya BJ, Cortessis VK, Schilperoort H, Kysh L, Matsuoka L, Yachimski P, Agrawal D, Gurudu SR, Jamil LH, Jue TL, Khashab MA, Law JK, Lee JK, Naveed M, Sawhney MS, Thosani N, Yang J, Wani SB. ASGE guideline on the role of endoscopy in the evaluation and management of choledocholithiasis. Gastrointest Endosc. 2019 Jun;89(6):1075–1105.e15. https://doi.org/10.1016/j.gie.2018.10.001. Epub 2019 Apr 9. PMID: 30979521.

9. Cotton PB, Feussner D, Dufault D, Cote G. A survey of credentialing for ERCP in the United States. Gastrointest Endosc. 2017 Nov;86(5):866–9. https://doi.org/10.1016/j.gie.2017.03.1530. Epub 2017 Mar 30. PMID: 28366439.
10. Cotton PB. Fading boundary between gastroenterology and surgery. J Gastroenterol Hepatol. 2000 Oct;15 Suppl:G34–7. https://doi.org/10.1046/j.1440-1746.2000.02263.x. PMID: 11100991.

Preface

I have been a consultant laparoscopic upper GI surgeon at London North West University Healthcare NHS Trust for the last 25 years and Mr Lalin Navaratne is a specialist registrar in upper GI surgery who has joined me in this project for the last six years. The single stage management of common bile duct stones has been a matter that has concerned me for the last 25 years. Since publication of NICE guidelines on gallstone disease in 2014, laparoscopic bile duct exploration (LBDE) has gained popularity within the UK and currently is considered the treatment of choice when local expertise is available. My experience in LBDE surgery commenced in 1998, and was the topic of a PhD, which I read at the University of Salamanca in 2019.

With my co-editor, Mr Lalin Navaratne, we have co-authored several publications which form the backbone of this text. Within the last two years, we began to amalgamate and condense all of the lessons learnt from a quarter century of pioneering this technique. This book accompanies our video *Laparoscopic Bile Duct Exploration* (DOI: https://doi.org/10.1007/978-3-030-95504-5; Online ISBN: 978-3-030-95504-5; Publisher: Springer) and *Laparoscopic Bile Duct Exploration: Problem-Based Learning Case Quiz* (DOI: https://doi.org/10.1007/978-3-030-95505-2; Online ISBN: 978-3-030-95505-2; Publisher: Springer), which provides detailed step-by-step instructions on how to undertake various techniques in LBDE. The content includes the indications of

LBDE, the materials and equipment required, and the surgical technique to successfully perform the procedure. This text is aimed to be a valuable reference guide for any surgeon who wishes to learn more about laparoscopic bile duct exploration.

London, UK   Alberto Isla
London, UK   Lalin Navaratne

Acknowledgments

From Alberto:
 To my wife Mireia and my daughters Andrea and Olivia.

From Lalin:
 Thank you to my parents for always supporting my dreams and my wife Susana and son Bosco for making these come true.

Contents

Chapter 1
History of Bile Duct Surgery

Alberto Martinez-Isla, María Asunción Acosta-Mérida, Lalin Navaratne, and Hutan Ashrafian

The First Cholecystectomy

The gallbladder has historically been considered an irreplaceable vital organ of the body associated with the fundamental elements of existence. The Sumerians and Babylonians considered vital for understanding life and utilised this organ (taken from ungulates) as part of their process to assess and predict life events as early as the fifth millennia BCE. By the time of Hippocrates (c.460–370 BCE), the gallbladder was

---

A. Martinez-Isla (✉) · L. Navaratne
Northwick Park and St Mark's Hospitals, London North West University Healthcare NHS Trust, London, UK
e-mail: a.isla@imperial.ac.uk; lalin.navaratne@doctors.org.uk

M. A. Acosta-Mérida
General Surgery Department, Hospital Universitario de Gran Canaria Doctor Negrín,
Las Palmas de Gran Canaria, Las Palmas, Spain

H. Ashrafian
The Department of Surgery and Cancer, St Mary's Hospital, Institute of Global Health Innovation, Imperial College London, London, UK

1

A. Martinez-Isla, L. Navaratne (eds.), *Laparoscopic Common Bile Duct Exploration*, In Clinical Practice,
https://doi.org/10.1007/978-3-030-93203-9_1

included in the underlying categorisation of the 'four humours' in health and therefore considered vitally important for life [1]. In 1508, Leonardo Da Vinci accurately identified and drew the cystohepatic triangle and was clear in presenting a known variant (in approximately 2% of individuals) where the cystic artery comes off the right hepatic artery (as opposed to the proper hepatic artery) [2].

In the nineteenth Century, Karl Langenbuch (1846–1901) (Fig. 1.1) was the first supporter of the theory that the gallbladder was a non-vital organ and that it could be removed without any problems for the patient, thereby introducing the concept of cholecystectomy. He studied medicine in Kiel and trained as a surgeon with Wilms, eventually becoming Chief of Surgery in Hospital Lazarus (Fig. 1.2). In that era, biliary disease was treated by physicians. The medical and surgical departments were close to each other which allowed him to observe the chronic and recurrent course of biliary disease. His first description of a cholecystectomy was in 1882. The original procedure was described in 1983 [3], and outlined the following concepts:

> Langenbuch suggested that the gallbladder was the place of the formation of stones, he avoided discussing its development in the bile duct. He also suspected that stones up to 1 cm would be able to pass into the duodenum [4].

> His plans of performing a cholecystectomy moved forward when he faced Mr H. a 40-year-old man who was one of the administrators of the hospital and that had been suffering from biliary colic with repeated cholecystitis and cholangitis since 1874; that rendered him a morphine addict and eventually killed him of secondary lymphangitis secondary to biliary sepsis. This experience and considering his assumption that the gallbladder was not a vital organ, made him start developing the technique of cholecystectomy working in cadaver; that brought him to the conclusion that this, with the ligation of the cystic duct, shouldn't be one of the most difficult procedures that require a laparotomy.

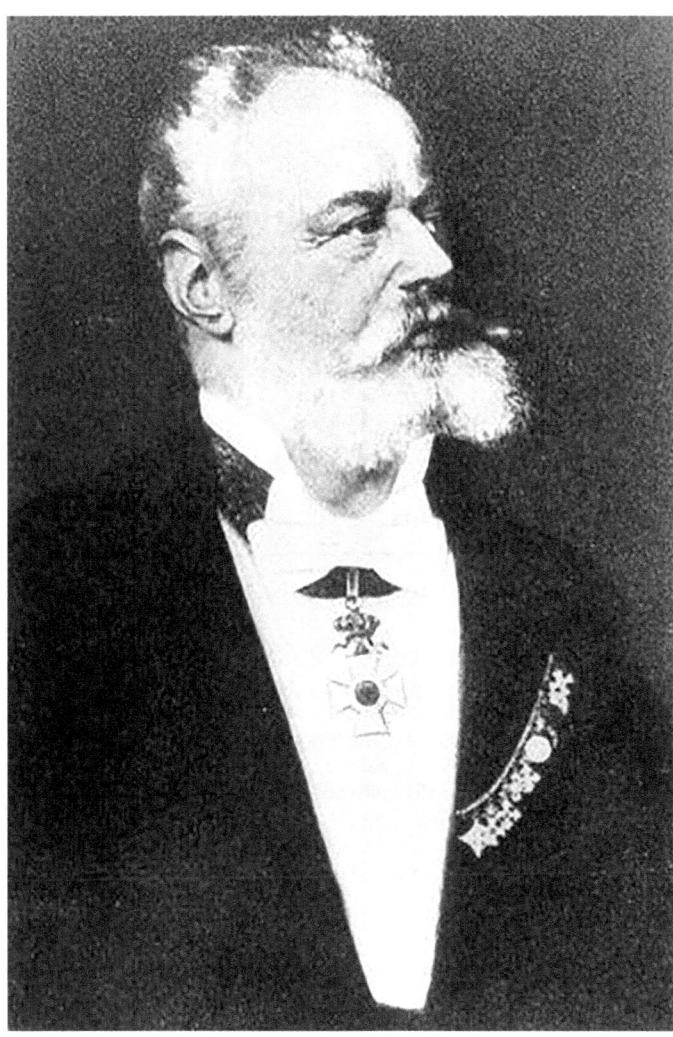

FIGURE 1.1 Dr. Karl Langenbuch

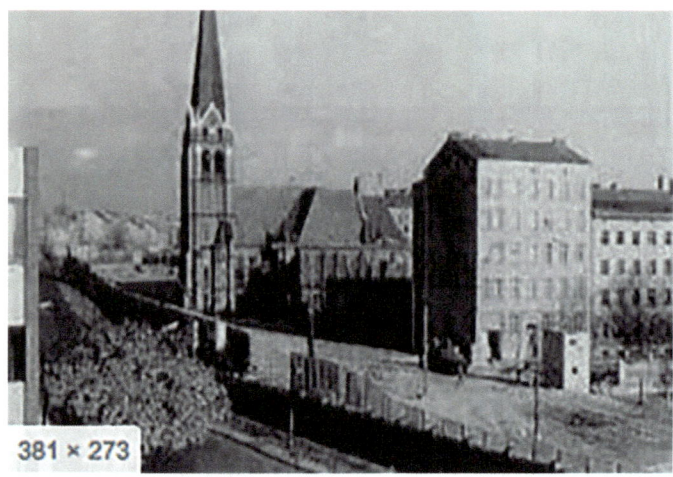

Figure 1.2 Hospital Lazarus

Following his work in cadavers he described the following technique:

> The laparotomy was T-shaped in the right upper quadrant with the vertical extension at the lateral border of the rectus muscle; he used a sponge to retract the small bowel and the colon under the abdominal wall. Then the hepatoduodenal ligament was tensioned by lifting the liver, helped with the retraction of the left hand of the assistant. The gallbladder was then freed of its adhesions and the cystic duct exposed, dissected, and ligated with silk 1–2 cm distal to the gallbladder; he was against using catgut because its absorbable nature. This should be followed by the dissection of the gallbladder from its bed and finally division of the cystic duct.

The ligation of the cystic artery was not mentioned, apart from this fact this technique doesn't differ much from the traditional open procedure that we all know.

Soon after he met Mr. D. a 43-year-old Court Secretary that presented in 1866 with biliary colic that was followed 3 years later by obstructive jaundice that lasted for 2 months. All those events made him lose 36 kg and suffer with lack of appetite nausea and persistent constipation. The days before the procedure he was suffering with daily attacks, leading to depression and requiring constant morphine. Facing this terrible picture Langenbuch offered Mr. D. performing a cholecystectomy which he accepted and therefore he was admitted at Lazarus on the tenth July 1882. Pre-operatively Mr. D was asked to rest in bed for 5 days and his bowels cleaned; on the 15th of July, helped by Dr. Martin and Professor Buch, Langenbuch proceeded with the cholecystectomy as he has previously described. The first post op night Mr. D. slept well, and at the time of the ward round he was smoking a cigar, on the third post-operative day he ate meat and mashed potatoes, the fourth day he spiked a temperature of 38.6° that disappeared the next day, and on the fifth and sixth days, he opened his bowels with loose stools, that greatly alleviated his symptoms. He got out of bed on the tenth day. By the time Langenbuch wrote the case up the patient had been well and without recurrence of all his symptoms.

As a reflection Langenbuch concluded that cholecystectomy *'was only indicated in the cases where both the patient and the surgeon had run out of patience though treatment by medical means, and therefore he considered it a last resource.'* He concluded his article analysing the risks of cholecystostomy *vs* cholecystectomy which *'with an adequate ligation of the cystic should be a more effective and less risky treatment for a diseased gallbladder'*. In 1884 in Philadelphia "Medical News" he published the editorial "Cholecystostomy and Cholecystectomy," concluding in favour of the former for having less risks [5]. This was contested by Lawson Tait (Fig. 1.3) a British surgeon who, initially described the cholecystectomy as absurd, but a year later changed his mind and wrote that it didn't seem to have a higher risk and completely prevents the recurrences [5] of biliary disease.

At that time the American opinion was mainly voiced by Musser & Keen, two surgeons from Philadelphia that wrote *'we should oppose to cholecystectomy, its only point would be preventing future formation of more calculi …..even in cases of severe inflammation, extraction of the stones and establishment of a fistula should be enough, so it doesn't make sense to*

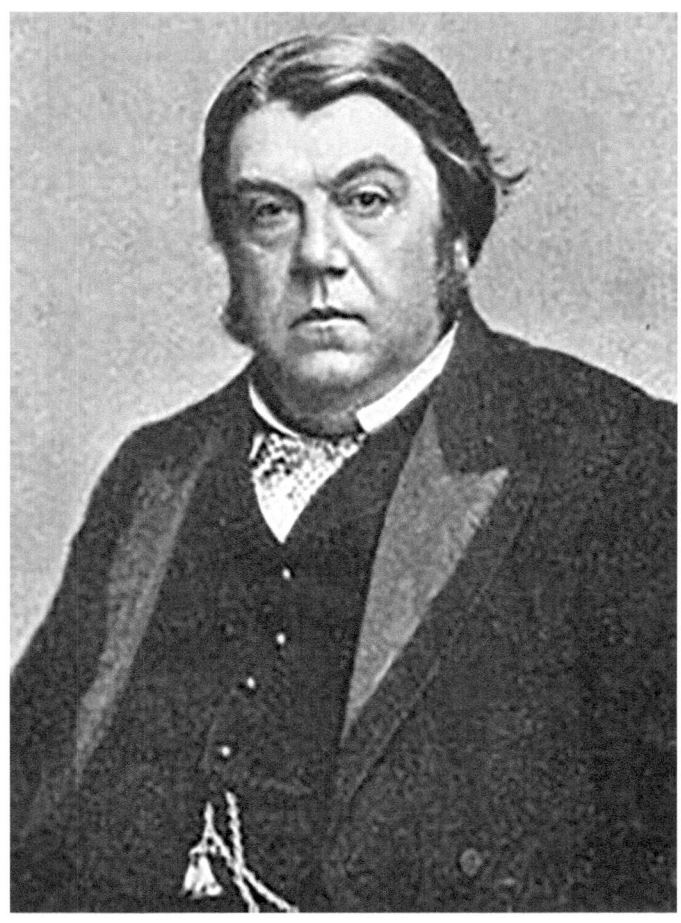

FIGURE 1.3 Dr. Lawson Tait

add the risk of the removal of the organ' [6]. This work was soon followed by Justus Ohage a German surgeon working in Minnesota who performed the first American cholecystec-tomy in 1886; he defined cholecystectomy as *'ideal that after curing the patient from his disease leaves him in the same situation that he was before'.* He reported a low mortality of one patient in 9 operations and he joined Langenbuch declaring the gallbladder as a non-essential organ. His paper was advanced in the sense that he discussed the indications of cholecystectomy and cholecystostomy, the former more indicated in young patients where the stone formations hasn't finished, the adhesions are manageable and the ducts patent [7]. William Worral Mayo, another surgeon also in Minnesota, often sent his sons William and Charles to watch Ohage operate, the Mayo family would be crucial in the ulterior expansion of cholecystectomy.

In the following 20 years cholecystectomy experienced an expansion through Europe and America with an important drop in its mortality. The Mayo family played an important role for that in America, and William Mayo in 1889 presented the experience of the hospital that bears his name, with just four cholecystectomies but encouraged to expand its practice [8], and 4 years later they had done 65 procedures. Charles Mayo in 1917 reported a mortality of less than 2%, but he would still defend the practice of cholecystostomies in patients with otherwise healthy gallbladders. In 1926, William Mayo published the Mayo Clinic experience showing large numbers, even 3 or 4 procedures a day [9], yet still mentioned performing some cholecystostomies. John Deaver, (1885–1931), famous for his retractor, besides this it seems that he performed more procedures in Philadelphia than anyone else before [10]. In his paper, he recommended that cholecystectomy should be performed by experience surgeons and generally when the gallbladder is not healthy, and it is likely the cause of infection.

In the 1920s it was accepted that cholecystectomy was the right approach, in the absence of severe inflammation that could jeopardise the dissection, this principle would continue valid during the following decades with a low mortality of 0.1–0.6% and bile duct injury 0.1–2% [11]. Figure 1.4 shows the increase in the number of cholecystectomies performed since 1894 with the reduction in its mortality.

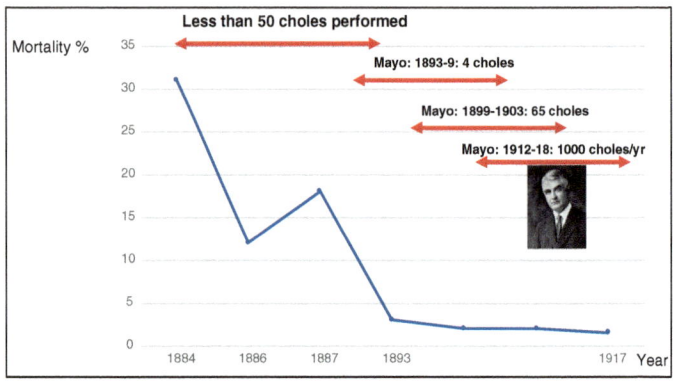

FIGURE 1.4 Evolution of number cholecystectomies performed and mortality (picture William James Mayo)

The First Choledochotomy

Now we will leave the cholecystectomy aside and we will see what happened with the management of the stones in the bile duct since the introduction of the cholecystectomy by Langenbuch. John Knowsley Thornton (1845–1904) (Fig. 1.5), on the ninth May 1889 in London, was the first to successfully perform the first choledochotomy. He started medicine late, aged 22, and after finishing he was appointed house officer to Lord Lister in Edinburgh, that marked in him a strong obsession with antisepsis and the excessive use of carbolic was often problematic. Before being a surgeon, he worked as General Practitioner in Northumberland and later he worked at the Samaritan Free Hospital, where surprisingly his main interest was ovariotomy. Nearly 7 years after the first cholecystectomy by Langenbuch, he performed the first choledochotomy and removed a large calculus. This was followed by the examination of the inside of the bile duct with a speculum. He presented his work at the Medical Society of London and this was later published in the Lancet [12, 13]. It is believed that this likely took place at the Samaritan Free

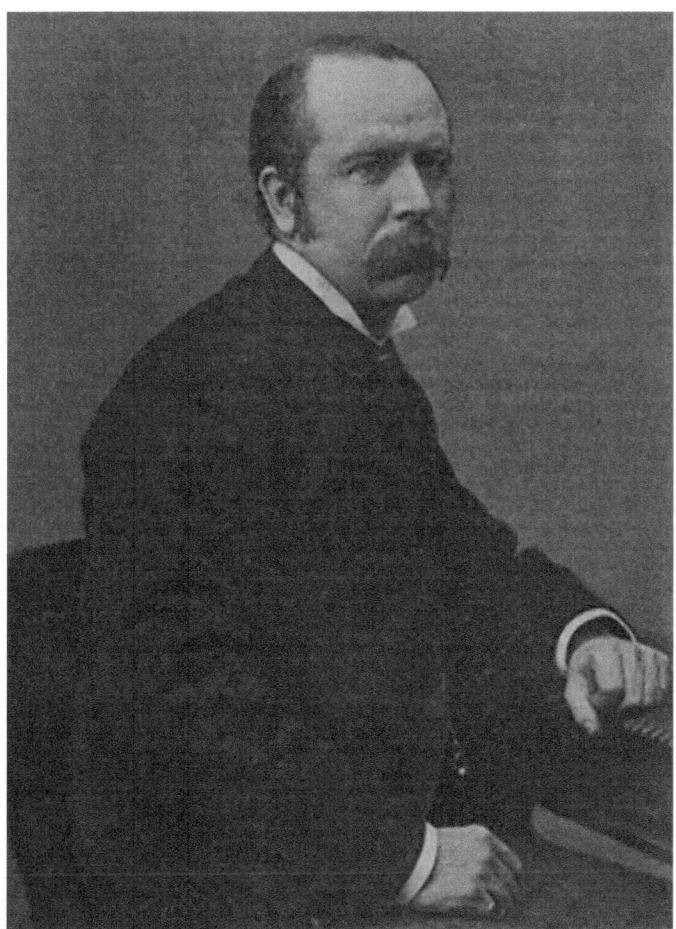

FIGURE 1.5 Dr. John K Thornton

Hospital. The original building is still in existence on London's Marylebone Road but sadly it is visibly decaying since it was abandoned nearly 25 years ago in 1997 (Fig. 1.6).

One year later, on 18th February 1890, Ludwing G. Courvoisier (1843–1918) (Fig. 1.7), who described the sign

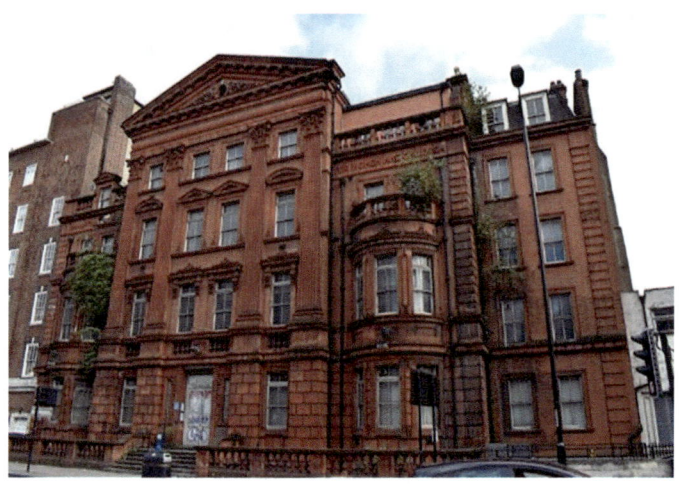

FIGURE 1.6 Samaritan Hospital, London

that bears his name, performed a choledochotomy in Riehen (Switzerland) [14], and finally Ludwing Rehn (1849–1930), better known for the first cardiac operation in the world [15], performed a combined cholecystectomy and bile duct exploration procedure. However, those were just isolated attempts to access the bile duct, and the techniques were not formally described and expanded upon until the early part of the twentieth century thanks to the work of Hans Kehr. Hans Kehr (1862–1916) (Fig. 1.8), who also described the T-tube, was instrumental in popularising bile duct surgery at beginning of the twentieth century.

Halstead, who operated on his mother who had choledocholithiasis in 1901, suggested that a method to diagnose the presence of stones in the bile duct was much needed. He would not guess that some years later he would suffer from bile duct stones. In 1919, he underwent a cholecystectomy that left him with retained stones, which ultimately developed into biliary fistula that resulted in his death in 1922 [14].

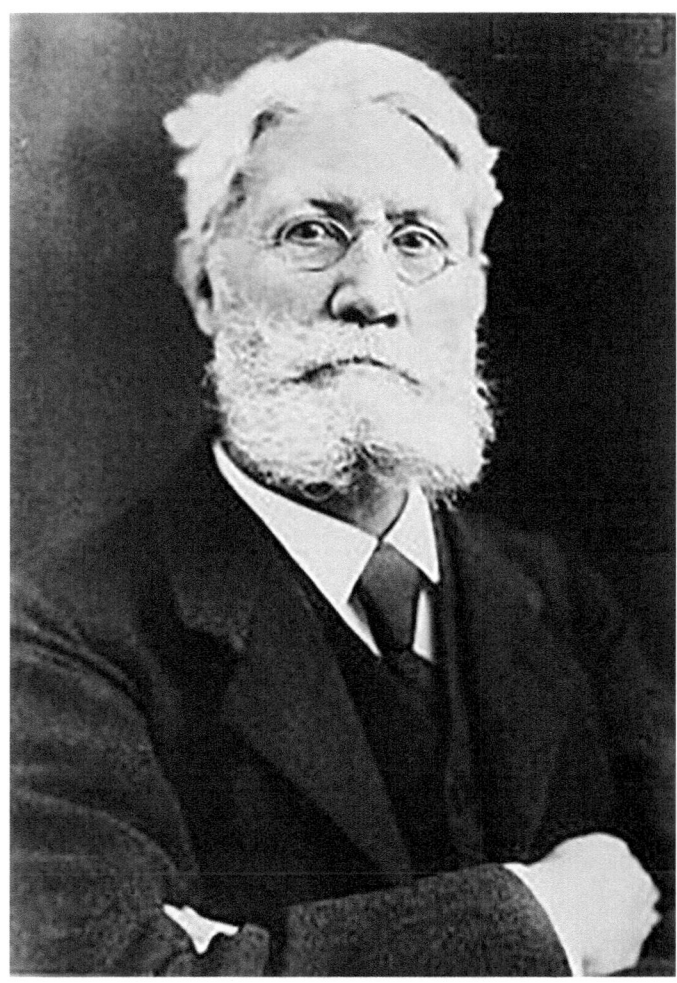

FIGURE 1.7 Dr. L G Courvoisier

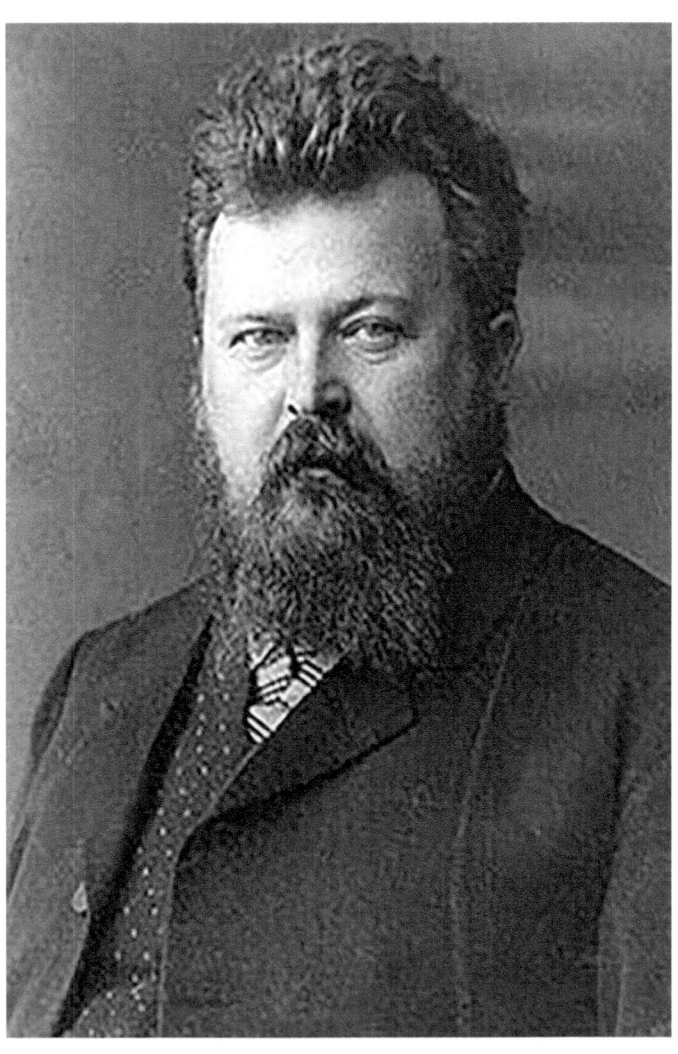

Figure 1.8 Dr. Hans Kehr

History of Common Bile Duct Imaging

As was suspected by Halstead, achieving an image of the bile duct was mandatory. Graham & Cole in 1924 introduced the cholecystogram to help to diagnose biliary disease, besides just with clinical history and physical examination [16]. The first radiological image of the biliary tree was accidentally obtained in 1918 by Reich, who injected bismuth and petrolate in order to define a fistula between the 10th and 11th rib, in one of his patients, Miss J de M, who had undergone pelvic surgery years before. After the injection, she presented with severe epigastric pain, followed by fever and jaundice the next day. An x-ray showed an opacified biliary tree draining into the duodenum. He treated her with heat, morphine, magnesium and warm olive oil injections through the tract [17].

This pioneering work may have paved the way for Pablo Luis Mirizzi (1893–1964) (Fig. 1.9) to develop the intraoperative cholangiogram (IOC). He was an Argentinian doctor, who graduated top of his class from Universidad de Cordoba in 1915. He underwent further training at the Mayo Clinic and in 1926 was appointed Professor of Surgery at Universidad Nacional de Cordoba. His main work was "Bile duct exploration during operation by injection of contrast substance". Amongst other achievements, he defined the Mirizzi syndrome. In 1959, the "*Société Internationale de Chirurgie*" in Munich nominated him president of the national congress. In 1938, he published his experience in "*Lancet*" [18]. Since 1931, he had performed intraoperative cholangiogram in all his cholecystectomies by injecting 3 cc of lipiodol® through the cystic, gallbladder or by direct puncture of the bile duct in 400 cases. In 55 patients with good drainage of the bile duct, he performed a primary closure. He emphasized the value of cholangiogram in order to bring the number of bile ducts explored to a minimum.

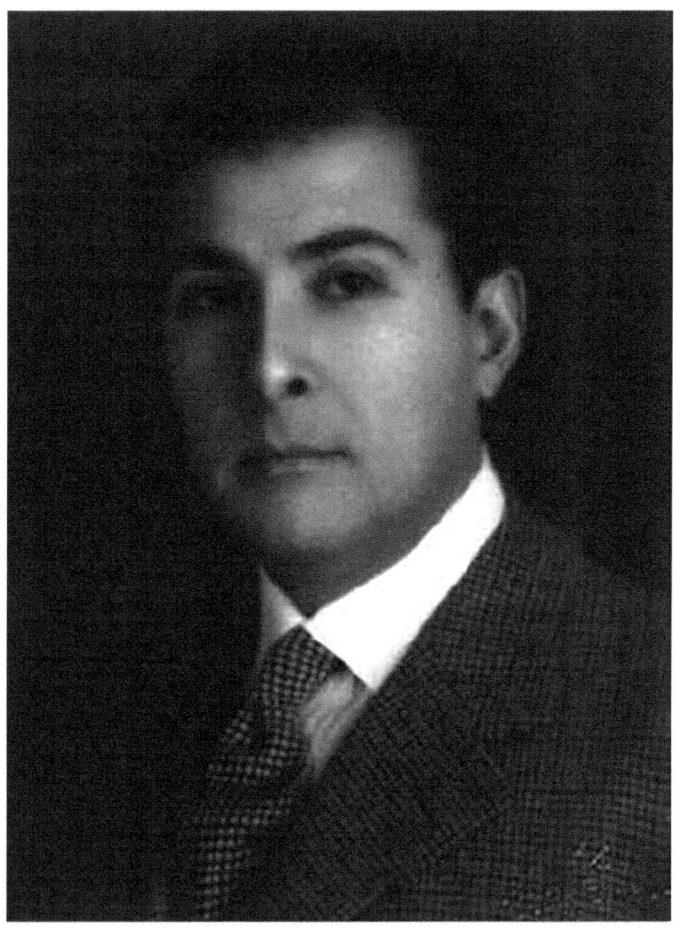

FIGURE 1.9 Dr. P L Mirizzi

Technique of Bile Duct Exploration in the 1960s and 1970s

The technique of bile duct exploration between 1960 and 1970 has been captured by Patel, as described in his book on surgical technique [19]. In the chapter *Surgery of the Bile Duct*, he described the silent forms of lithiasis, without clinical or radiological manifestations. When he described bile duct exploration, he did so with a diagnostic rather than therapeutic aim, and he classified it into: manual, manometric/radiologic and instrumental transcystic. Surprisingly, he gave priority to the diagnostic manometric over the radiologic, because he believed this can give information about the sphincter of Oddi and allow its classification into: normal, hypertonic and hypotonic. He also postulated that use of these diagnostic methods could abolish the presence of post-cholecystectomy syndrome. He also mentioned that the transcystic instrumental exploration is preferred by the Anglo-Saxon authors, which is performed after dilatation of the cystic with Bengolea forceps, using Bake's dilators introduced into the duodenum. In the case of an unobstructed duct, this can be palpated through the duodenal wall (Fig. 1.10). If the presence of a stone was suspected then a choledochotomy would be required (Figs. 1.11 and 1.12), and even in some cases a transduodenal approach with sphincteroplasty might have been needed (Fig. 1.13). He described the indications of performing a choledochotomy between the two extremes: on one end of the spectrum those patients who have an obvious obstruction with a dilated duct and the other end of the spectrum those with non-dilated bile ducts with good passage. He defined the difficulty of choledochotomy as being inversely proportional to its diameter and presence of inflammation. He recommended opening the bile duct distal to the insertion the cystic duct, principles that are still valid to this day. The choledochotomy was performed longitudinally with a knife between 2 stay sutures (Fig. 1.11) and it was followed by the introduction of the stone forceps after some degree of Kocherisation had been achieved (Fig. 1.12). Once the duct had been explored, in order to check that no residual stones had been left behind, Patel recommended matching the number of stones extracted to the number present on the cholangiogram. Surprisingly, he didn't advocate performing a completion cholangiogram.

In the textbook, choledochoscopy is initially described, using a rigid Wildegans instrument with a 120° angle (Fig. 1.14).

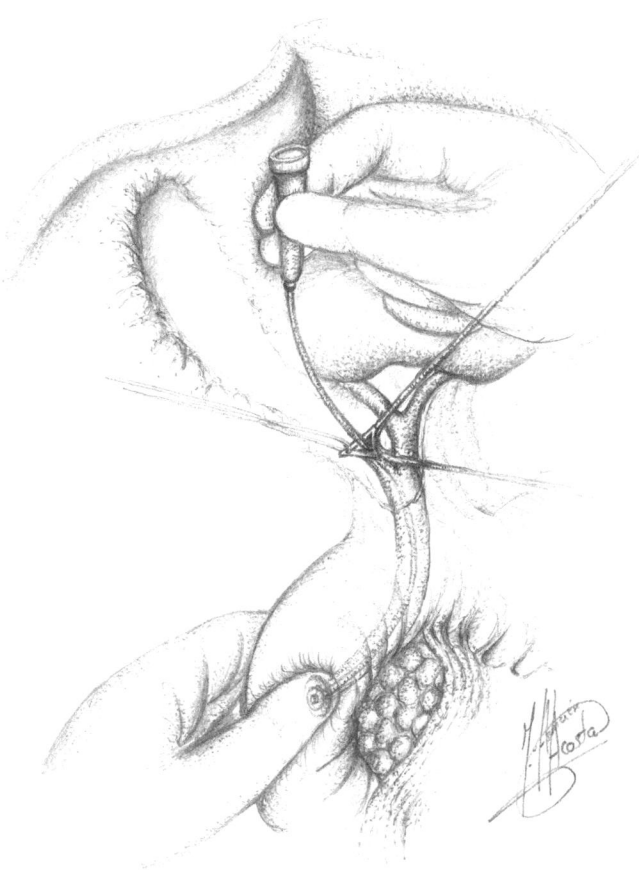

Figure 1.10 Transcystic

This instrument appeared to be valuable in obtaining a proximal view of the bile duct and the intra-hepatic bifurcation but not very useful for examination of the distal duct. We would have to wait until 1965 for the first flexible choledochoscope to be available (American Cystoscope Makers Inc., Southborough, MA, USA). In 1973, Longland used this scope for the first reported flexible choledochoscopy in the UK [20]. Longland performed 37 choledochoscopies in 35 patients,

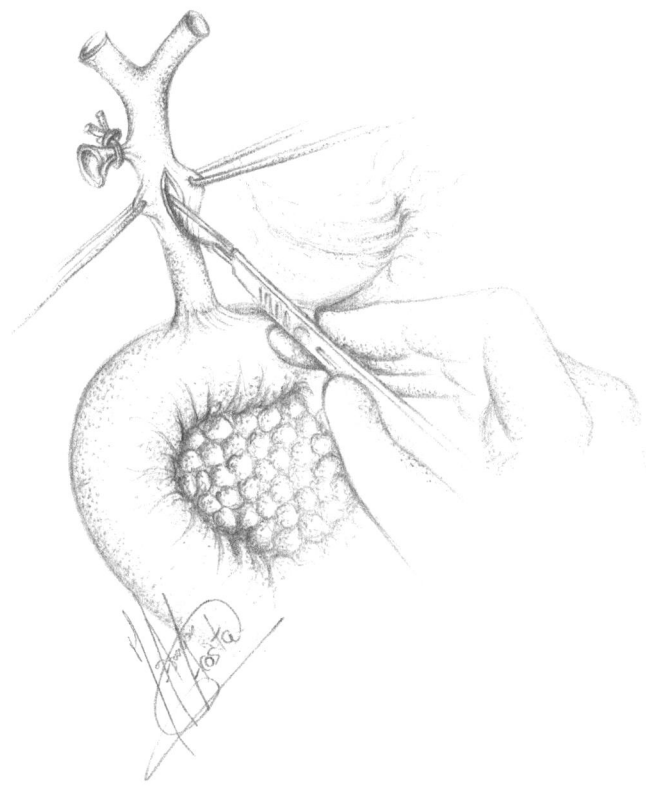

FIGURE 1.11 Choledochotomy

mainly to clarify dubious cholangiograms. He described his technique and experience with 35 patients. He found stones on 26 occasions in 24 patients with 11 blank examinations (30%). The stones were initially extracted blindly, which was then followed by choledochoscopy. In 24 patients, 11 had residual stones and 13 were clear, therefore the CBD was closed over a T-tube. In 11 patients with residual stones, the extraction failed in two, therefore a choledochoduodenostomy was performed. Longland's report was very advanced for its time, and he also recommended primary closure of the

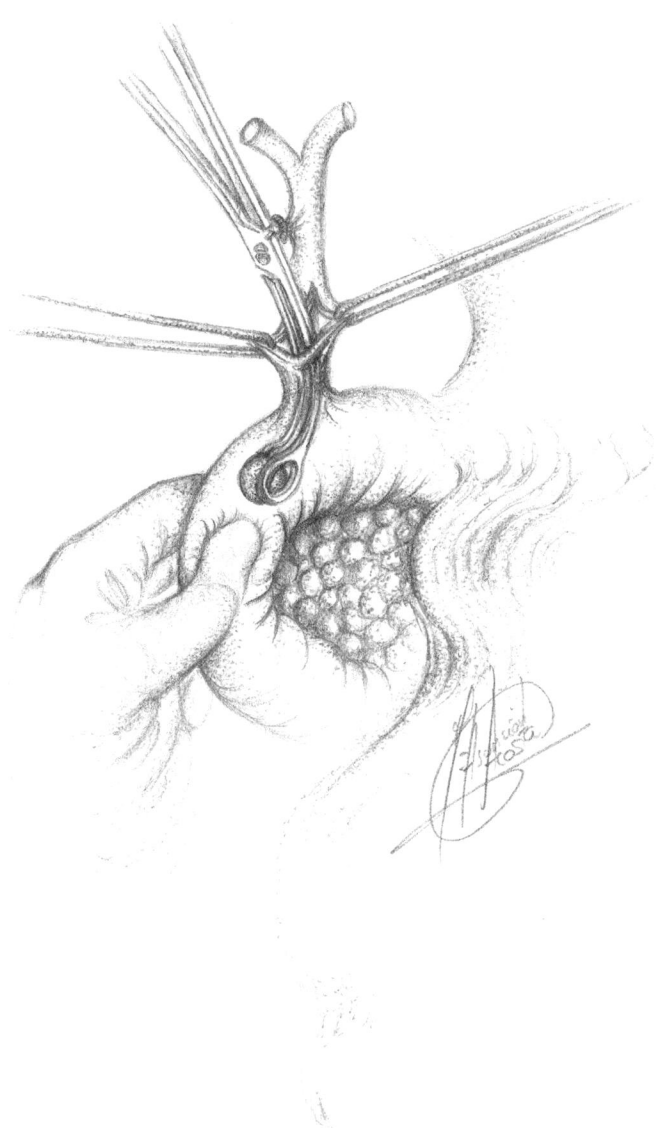

FIGURE 1.12 Transductal exploration

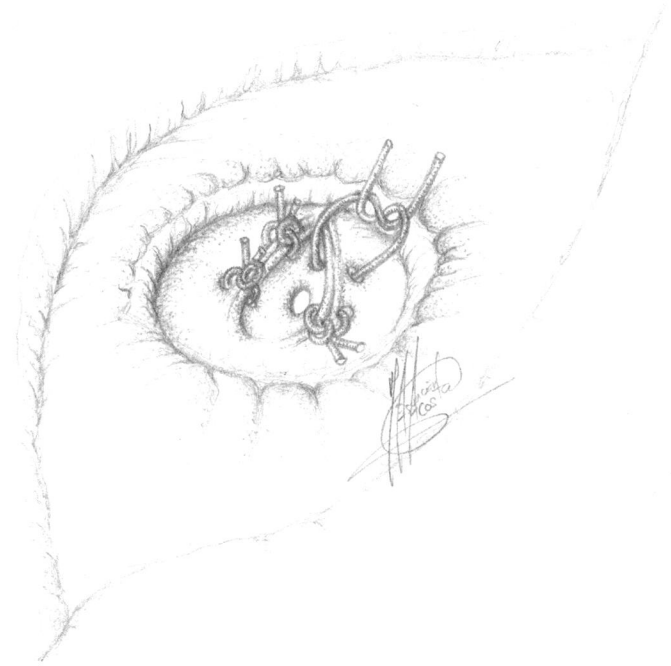

FIGURE 1.13 Transduodenal sphincteroplasty

bile duct but only exceptionally, when there was a healthy duct combined with very good distal drainage. He routinely recommended closure of the bile duct over a T-tube, as described in Fig. 1.15. At that time, he used vascular silk or catgut 00 or 000, sometimes closing the peritoneum over it.

The Arrival of Endoscopic Retrograde Cholangiopancreatography (ERCP)

Much of the techniques previously described was referenced between 1959–1973. In 1968, biliary surgery was about to change forever with the reporting of the first endoscopic cannulation of the papilla by McCune and colleagues [21].

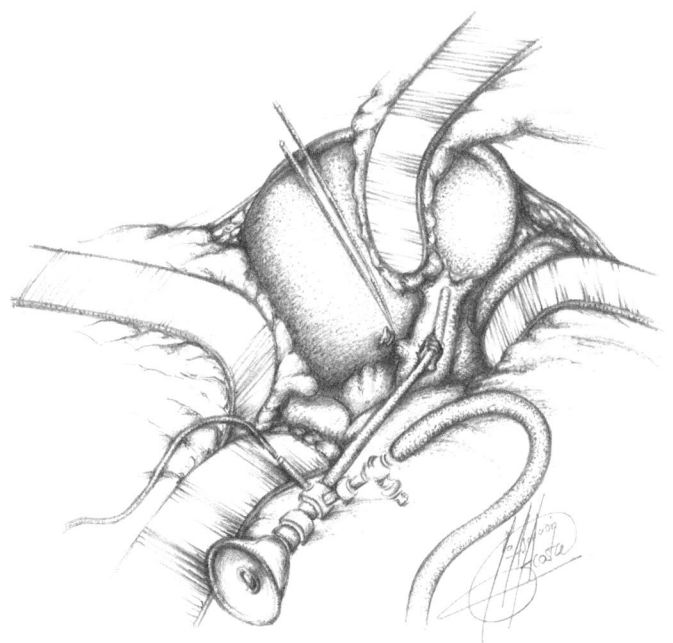

FIGURE 1.14 Choledochoscope of Wildegans

McCune's work was well received, because at the time, there was no accurate diagnostic imaging for the pancreas, which had previously been achieved by indirect imaging. His work was centred on the non-operative injection of radiopaque material into the pancreatic duct through the ampulla of Vater. The first time that this was achieved was in 1965 by Simon and Rabinov [22]. McCune et al., attached a cannula housing onto an Eder fibreoptic duodenoscope. It had a light source and a mobile tip helped by a balloon and controlled from the handle. They used Valium and Demerol as sedative medication and injected 5 cc of 50% Hypaque through the cannula. They reported a 50% cannulation rate and no mortality. In 1972, Peter Cotton reported his experience with 63 patients achieving an 80% cannulation success rate [23]. He used Olympus JFB (Figs. 1.16 and 1.17) and Machida FDS

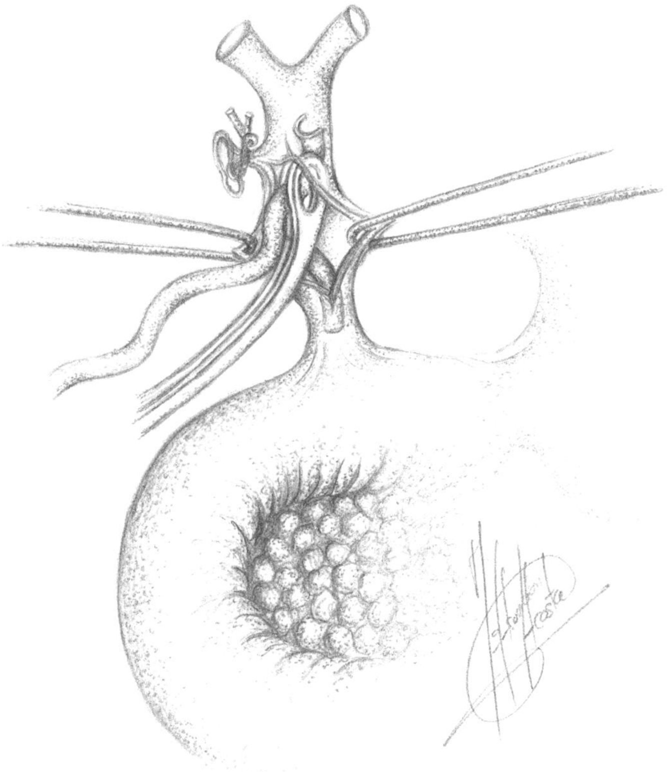

FIGURE 1.15 Insertion of T-tube

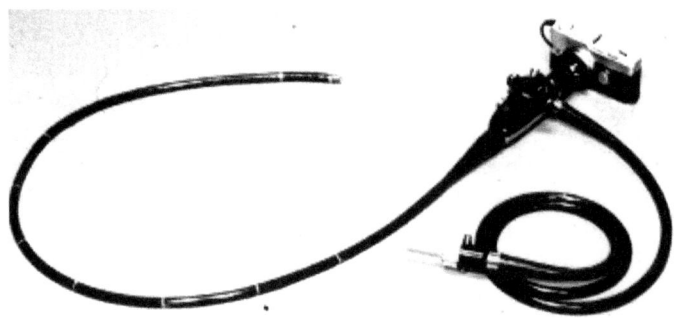

FIGURE 1.16 Cotton's Olympus scope (Courtesy of Dr. Peter Cotton)

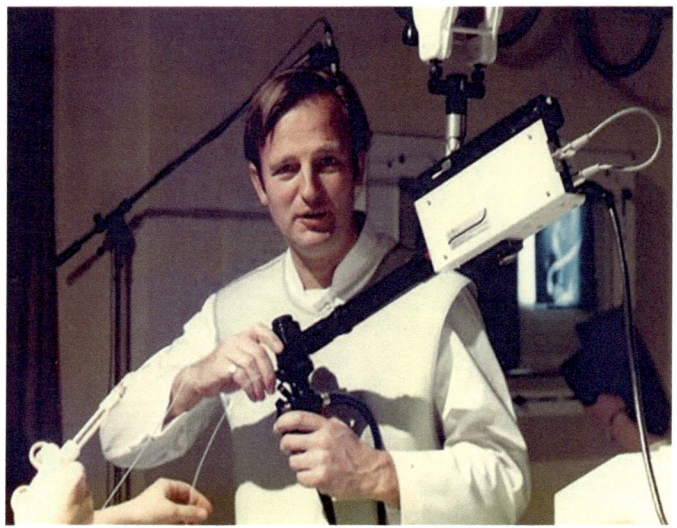

FIGURE 1.17 Dr. Peter Cotton at work (Courtesy of Dr. Peter Cotton)

scopes, the latter difficult to get outside of Japan. In his publication, he quoted a cost of £2500 for this instrument! Cotton described ERCP as a teamwork between the endoscopist, the radiologist, the interventional radiologist and the surgeon (Fig. 1.18). The procedure was performed with the patient in a left semi-prone position and his endoscope did not have the balloon as described by McCune [21], but did have lateral vision. Following the procedure, he recommended 36 h of inpatient observation. Interestingly, he mentioned pancreatitis and Australia antigen positive as contraindications. He reported that one third of patients will be successfully cannulated without difficulty and a cholangiogram can be achieved by just introducing the cannula 5 mm. At that time, the cannulation rates were 75–96%.

Cotton's work initially was mainly aimed at diagnosis and surprisingly in his indications, he didn't mention choledocholithiasis, with the focus being mainly pancreatic disease. Cotton describes ERCP as difficult to learn and perform, but

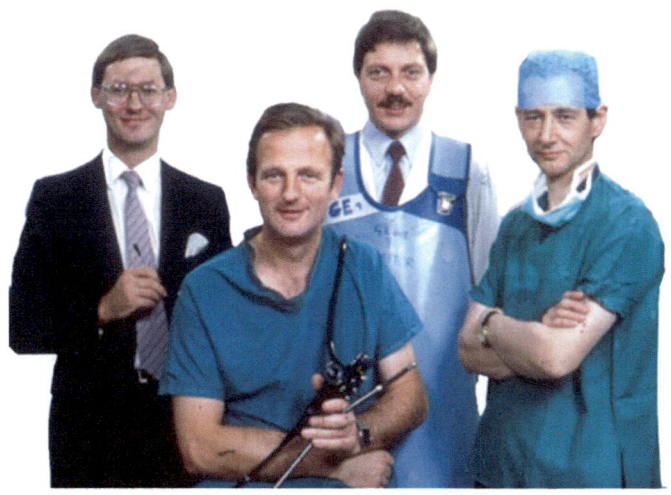

FIGURE 1.18 Dr. Peter Cotton with radiology colleagues and surgical colleague Mr. Russel (Courtesy of Dr. Peter Cotton)

he stills prioritises it against transhepatic cholangiogram. His work didn't pass unnoticed by the surgeons, and the President of the Royal College of Surgeons of England at the time, Lord Rodney Smith, at the end of one of his talks said the College should charge corkage on each stone removed by a gastroenterologist. It was Cotton who coined the acronym ERCP, that was subsequently officially approved at the Mexico City World congress [24].

In 1974, Kawai et al. in Japan [25] and Classem and Demling [26] in Germany simultaneously report the first endoscopic sphincterotomy (Figs. 1.19 and 1.20). Only Kawai's report was published in English. His group described performing two successful endoscopic sphincterotomies and extraction of stones in two patients and failure of the technique in another patient. They used the same technique for polypectomy but applied to the ampulla of Vater. With the electrode inserted into the working channel of the Olympus duodenoscope, the papilla was cannulated as per cholangio-pancreatography. The technical failure in one patient was

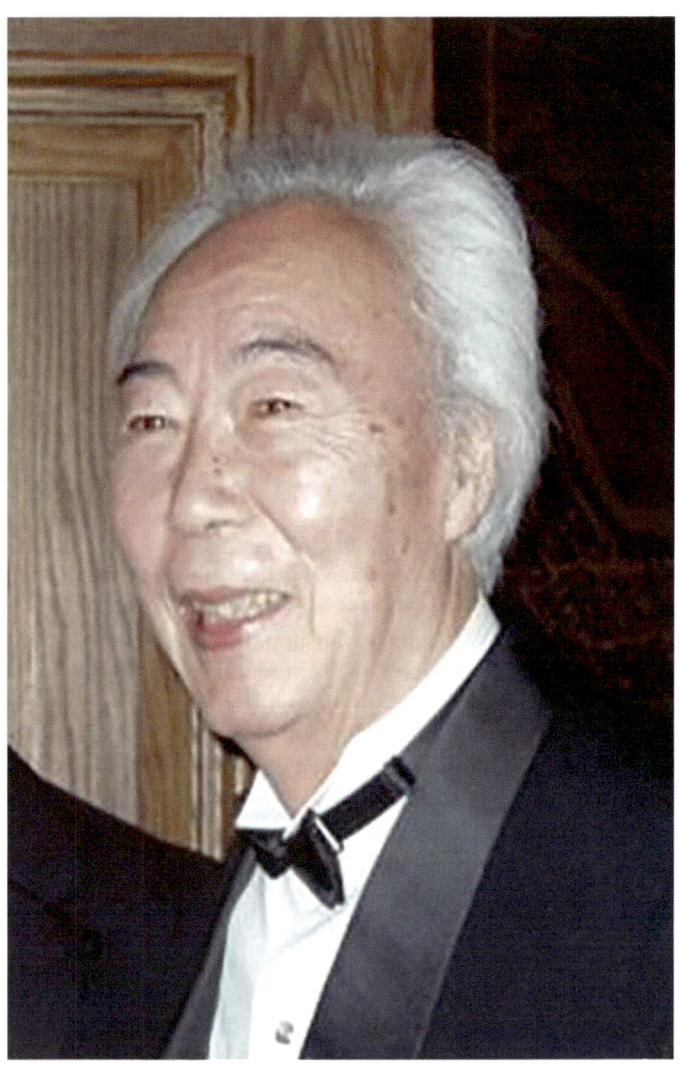

FIGURE 1.19 Kawai (Courtesy of Dr. Peter Cotton)

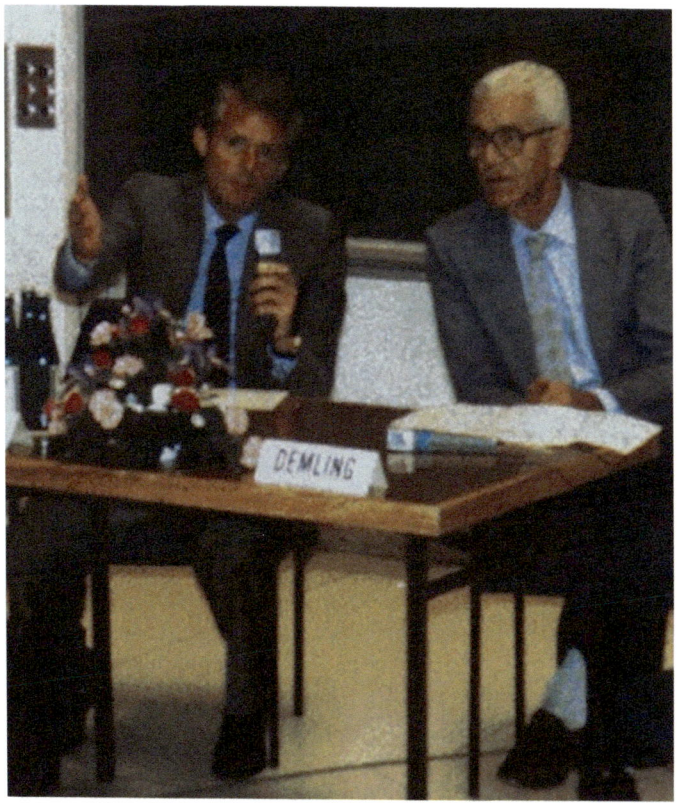

FIGURE 1.20 Classen and Demling (Courtesy of Dr. Peter Cotton)

because of the inability to cannulate the ampulla. The two successful patients were a 29-year-old male that presented with painful jaundice, the diagnosis was made when the stone was seen protruding on a barium meal and confirmed on a transhepatic cholangiogram. As planned the papilla was cut open with the electrode and a control endoscopy performed a week later confirmed extraction of the stone. The second patient was a 48-year-old female with a retained stone after a cholecystectomy and bile duct exploration with a T-tube. Sphincterotomy and stone extraction were successful and

T-tube cholangiography confirmed it. Kawai finished his article without knowing that a new era in the treatment of ductal stones was just born.

Approach to Common Bile Duct Stones in the 1980s

Until the end of the 1980s, the management of ductal stones changed very little. The approach to ductal stones at that time was captured in Professor Blumgart's 'Surgery of the Liver and Biliary Tract' textbook. In the chapter dedicated to cholecystectomy, JM Ham described the technique, which differs very little from the initial description by Langenbuch [27], but reported a lesser morbidity and mortality. Ham emphasised the importance of the dissection of Calot's triangle (Fig. 1.21), what later would be defined as the 'critical view of safety', as a safeguard to decrease the incidence of bile duct injuries. He also recommended the use of absorbable material and he challenged the manoeuvre of closing the peritoneum on the gallbladder bed and the use of drains. All those principles could be applied to today's standard laparoscopic cholecystectomy technique.

In the chapter dedicated to bile duct stones [28], Girard and Legros described manual palpation or cholangiography as the most common methods to detect ductal stones. They associated the addition of a bile duct exploration to the cholecystectomy with a 3-to-7-fold increase in morbidity and mortality. They therefore recommended surgeons to have a high index of suspicion before embarking upon bile duct exploration. When it was needed, they advised performing the choledochotomy at the supraduodenal portion of the bile duct, and if necessary, to complement this with a transduodenal approach in case of distal impacted stones. They also recommended performing a completion cholangiogram and they introduced the concept of choledochoscopy.

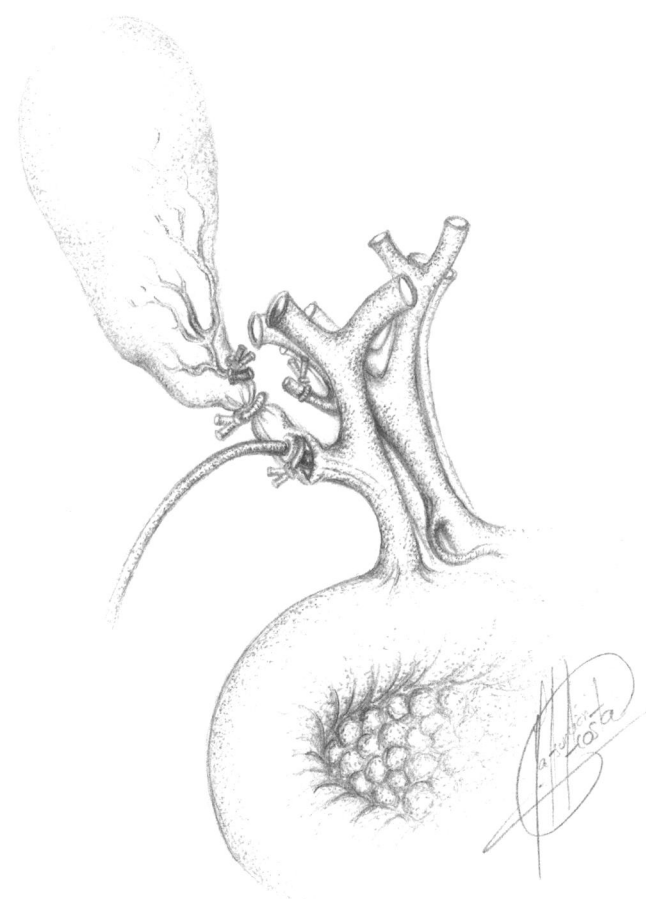

FIGURE 1.21 Dissection of Calot's triangle

They recommended closure of the choledochotomy over a T-tube, at least 14F, to allow its use in case of retained stones. Their indications for bilioenteric anastomosis were:

1. Multiple stones, elderly patients and dilated ducts
2. Large stones in dilated ducts

3. Failure to remove intrahepatic stones
4. Papillary stenosis
5. Distal impacted stones

Table 1.1 shows the Girard (819 ductal explorations) as well as McSherry's (1371 ductal explorations) data, together with other authors [28]. Our own experience to date since 1998 is nearly 500 laparoscopic explorations. Some of the authors only found stones in 50% of the of explorations, and their approach to the bile duct was not laparoscopic transcystic 3 mm choledochoscopy, as we aim to do today. The same author refers to the presence of retained stones after bile duct exploration in 83 patients, three of those requiring a third

TABLE 1.1 Incidence of CBD stones in patients with gallstones (from Girard RM)

Authors	Total cases of gallstones	CBD Explorations %	Positive explorations %	Overall incidence of CBS stones
Way et al. 1972	952	21	65	14
Kakos et al. 1972	753	25	62	15
McSherry & Glenn 1980	8971	15.6	59.7	9.3
Hampson et al. 1981	2889	15	51	7.8
Doyle et al. 1984	4000	22	52.5	11.5
Lygidakis et al. 1983	3710	11.6	80	9.4
Coelho et al. 1984	908	21	72	14.9
Girard 1988	7436	11	71.8	7.9

operation. This suggests that in 1984, the management of ductal stones was surgical, despite of ERCP being an established technique. Girard concluded saying that the success of bile duct exploration is *'exploring all and only those patients with choledocholithiasis'* and that the most reliable method to confirm that the bile duct is clear are the completion cholangiogram and choledochoscopy.

Since the first report of choledochoscopy in 1973, very little happened until Ashby, who in 1985 published his work in the *British Journal of Surgery* [29]. He described an impressive 150 patient series over an 8-year period (127 with ductal stones). He realised that the technique for stone extraction was not quite there, and in fact it would take a few more years to develop. He mentioned the important role of palpation during bile duct exploration and emphasised the important problem caused by retained stones, which became the main focus of his work. He used and described the Olympus CHF-10 reusable choledochoscope, which allowed sterilization by immersion. He reported his technique of choledochoscopy through a right subcostal incision extended over the midline, and like Longland he described the concept of the hepatic carina as the choledochoscopic view of the bifurcation of the intra-hepatic ducts due to its resemblance to the bronchial bifurcation (Fig. 1.22). Ashby described the use of balloons, baskets and forceps, and reported a 41% rate of negative choledochoscopy. This is because when CBD stones were suspected, he would go directly to choledochoscopy, rather than performing an intraoperative cholangiogram. This has similarities to our current practice as we have a low threshold for direct choledochoscopy when using a laparoscopic transcystic approach with a 3 mm choledochoscope. Ashby pioneered primary closure of choledochotomy, with a 2% rate of prolonged bile leaks, and 'a number' showing some bile in the drain for a few days. He also stressed the difficulty of achieving a waterproof closure, which is not surprising considering he used 000 catgut. Finally, he concluded that blind exploration and extraction of stones should be avoided, the surgeon should be able the inspect the inside of the ducts and that choledochoscopy does not seem to increase morbidity.

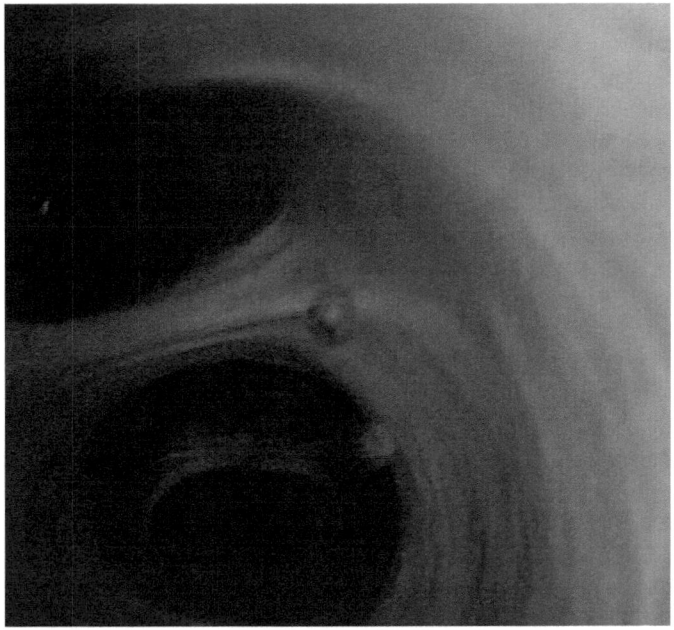

FIGURE I.22 Intra-hepatic bifurcation

The Revolution in the 1990s: Laparoscopic Cholecystectomy and Bile Duct Exploration

At the same time that Blumgart's book was printed in 1988, and just 3 years after Ashby's work on choledochoscopy, a revolution was brewing in the surgical world: the laparoscopic cholecystectomy. The pioneers of this new technique are listed in Table 1.2. Professor Erich Mühe (Fig. 1.23) from Böblingen on 12th September 1985 became the first surgeon to perform a laparoscopic cholecystectomy with a lateral view scope in Berlin. However, his work was never published in the English language which is why Mouret of France, is often credited as the first person to perform this operation. Reynolds described the technique and instruments used during the first laparoscopic cholecystectomy [30]. The three

TABLE 1.2 The pioneers of laparoscopic cholecystectomy

Name	Country	Date
Mühe	Germany	September 1985
Mouret	France	March 1987
Dubois	France	April 1988
McKernan and Saye	USA	June 1988
Reddick and Olsen	USA	September 1988
Berci	Australia	September 1988
Perissat	France	November 1988
Cuschieri	UK	February 1989

most important, basic instruments used for the first laparoscopic cholecystectomy were the laparoscope (used by the gynaecologists for many years), the haemoclip® (Weck-Reynolds pistol grip clip applier) and the scissors (Weck-Reynolds pistol grip scissors). In 1972, Weck & Co developed instruments for Reynolds. These were to be used in open surgery to ligate ducts and blood vessels. Reynolds then started to perform minimally invasive cholecystectomies using these instruments through a pararectal incision because this seemed to be tolerated better than the conventional open cholecystectomy. Mühe used the same instruments for his first laparoscopic cholecystectomy in 1985, which he confirmed in a personal communication to Reynolds in January 1998.

In 1972, Erich Mühe was assistant to Professor Gerd Hegeman, and returning from a congress where he saw the advantages of laparoscopy, convinced him to introduce laparoscopy in their surgical clinic. In 1980, Semm performed the first laparoscopic appendicectomy [31] and fascinated by his work, Mühe began to develop the idea of laparoscopic cholecystectomy. In 1982, Mühe was appointed Chief of Surgery at the Böblingen County Hospital in Bîblingen and in 1984 he designed an endoscope with side-viewing optics (the 'galloscope'), which was used to perform the first laparoscopic

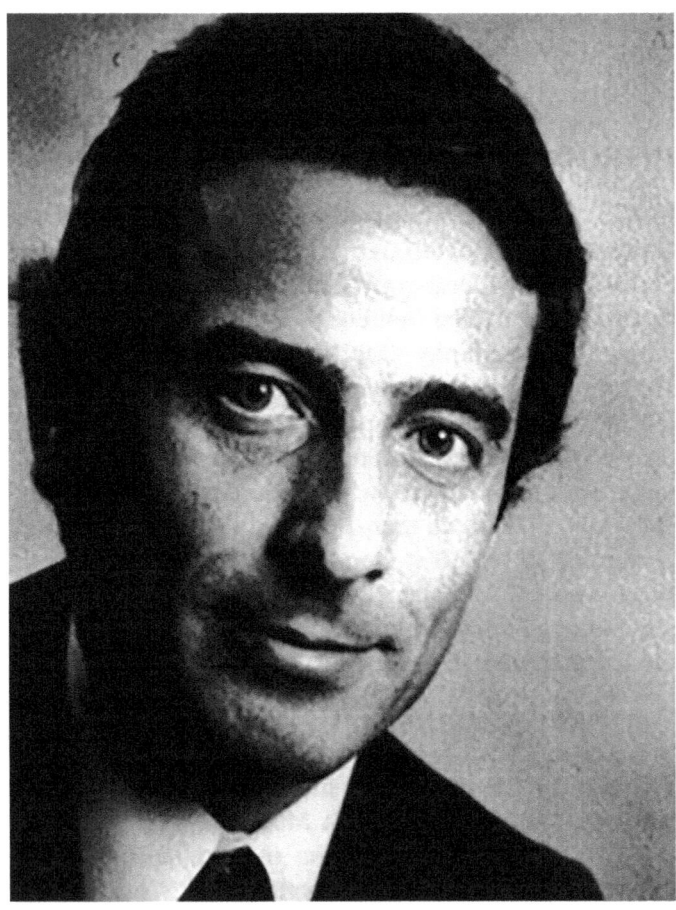

FIGURE 1.23 Dr. Erich Mühe

cholecystectomy. Mühe published his work in Endoscopy [32] as follows: *'The first endoscope constructed and used by ourselves ('Galloscope') had side-viewing optics, and an instrumentation channel with valves, a light conductor and a duct for the establishment of continuous pneumoperitoneum by the Veress needle technique; the endoscope was introduced through the umbilicus into the peritoneal cavity. For the insertion, we* *used a sharp mandrel within a trocar sleeve. After removal of the mandrel, a trap valve was ejected from the inner wall of the tube to seal off escaping CO_2. When the gallbladder was removed under optical control through the endoscope, the top of the endoscope had to be taken off. However, the gallbladder could also be removed through the trocar sleeve.'* From 1986, Mühe presented his work at the German Surgical Society on several occasions, but this was received with scepticism. Perhaps America would have been a better audience, but only 7% of the 342 articles that he published between 1965 and 1973 were written in English. Furthermore, he submitted an article to the *American Journal of Surgery* in 1990 which was rejected because the English language was substandard. However, the wheels were already set in motion and the procedure soon would extend across Europe, but this time as Litynski mentions in his book, led by a French surgeon, Phillipe Mouret and the 'French Connection' [31, 33].

In 1987, Mouret was in Lyon performing a gynaecological operation on a woman who also suffered from gallstones. When he directed the laparoscope upwards, he saw the gallbladder, and decided (not without difficulty), to perform a cholecystectomy. Francois Dubois, another French surgeon, learned about Mouret's work from a theatre nurse, Claire Jeaupitre, who had previously worked with Mouret in Lyon. They met soon after at the Paris Hilton in December 1987 as Mouret happened to be visiting Paris for a gynaecological meeting. Dubois, an enthusiast of the mini-cholecystectomy, was convinced by Mouret of the advantages of the laparoscopic cholecystectomy but his self-acknowledged lack of laparoscopic experience meant that he converted his first cases into open surgery: '*At the very beginning I was not skilled enough to finish this procedure in the endoscopie way. The first operations I always began laparoscopically, but I finished the procedure using laparotomy. Finally, it worked! My first fully laparoscopic cholecystectomy was done at the end of April 1988.*' Dubois published his early experience of laparoscopic cholecystectomy in 36 patients in the *Annals of Surgery* [34]. During this time, Jacques Perissat of Bordeaux,

France, was heavily invested in extracorporeal shock wave lithotripsy (ESWL) for gallbladder disease, but its poor results lead him to develop a technique of laparoscopic assisted intracorporeal lithotripsy via cholecystotomy. After attending one of Dubois lectures, he was given the idea of performing cholecystectomy in place of cholecystotomy, and became the third person who would help to expand laparoscopic cholecystectomy across Europe. He published their groups initial experience in *Endoscopy* and *Surgical Endoscopy* [35]. Perissat reported that he performed an intravenous cholangiogram the day before surgery and for the operation he used two 10 mm and two 5 mm ports, a 10 mm laparoscope with a cold light source, and a CO_2 insufflator with a pressure monitor. The instruments were diathermy scissors, atraumatic graspers and a titanium-clip applier. Pneumoperitoneum was created with a Veress needle and this was followed by insertion of the supraumbilical 10 mm trocar and the other 3 trocars (Fig. 1.24). Once the cholecystectomy was completed, the gallbladder was removed through the umbilical incision. Surprisingly, his description did not mention either the critical view or the systematic dissection of the hilum. He attempted the procedure in 39 patients and 3 (8%) required conversion to open surgery. He had two main complications: a patient with bleeding who required mini-laparotomy and another laparotomy for biliary peritonitis. In the 3 months since he reviewed the proofs of his paper until its final publication, he operated on a further 220 patients, the last 180 being uncomplicated. The new era of laparoscopic cholecystectomy was born that would change the face of biliary surgery forever.

With the expansion of the technique there was an increase in the number of publications on both sides of the Atlantic, including Karl Zucker's (Baltimore, Maryland, USA) book published in 1991 [36]. The textbook portrayed the American perspective on laparoscopy and 98% of the authors were American. Surprisingly, it didn't mention Professor Erich Mühe in the development of the procedure and it was a basic book describing the principles of laparoscopy including

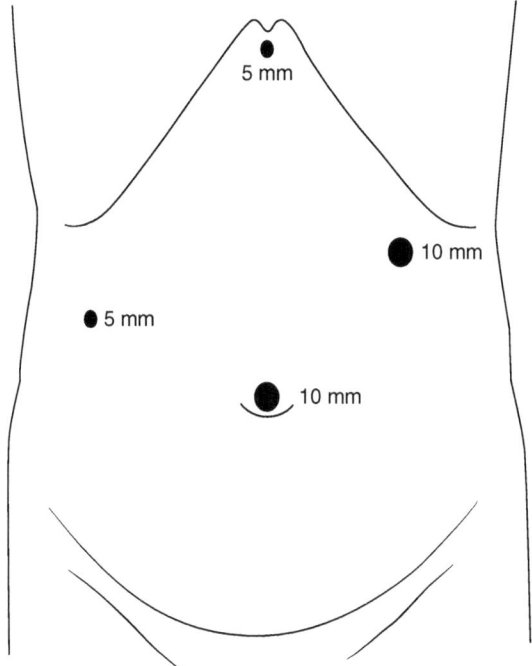

FIGURE 1.24 Port placement: French position

instruments, energy devices, anaesthesia, indications (cancer staging, cholecystectomy, appendicectomy, pelvic lymphadenectomy, vagotomy and inguinal hernia) and complications. Unlike the French authors, they recommended the American technique (Fig. 1.25), the main differences being that no ports are placed on the left side of the abdomen and the surgeon stands to the left of the supine patient. The textbook included a chapter on choledocholithiasis [37]. The use of intraoperative cholangiogram was mainly to prevent bile duct injuries and it was advised against laparoscopic management of the stones found. It seems that the main reason to recommend performing an intraoperative cholangiogram was to provide legal cover against bile duct injuries that could happen during a procedure that was in its infancy. Therefore, the authors'

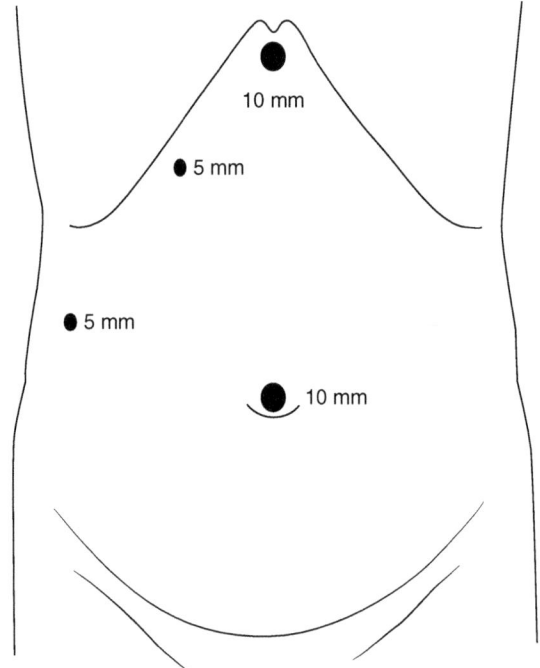

FIGURE 1.25 Port placement: American position

recommendation was to perform exhaustive screening for CBD stones pre-operatively. If there were CBD stones present, the CBD was to be cleared prior to laparoscopic cholecystectomy with pre-operative ERCP. Finding ductal stones during the cholecystectomy was considered a failure of pre-operative screening. However, in this scenario, it was recommended to convert to open surgery or alternatively perform post-operative ERCP, preferably the former because the latter could also fail and condemn the patient to a second laparotomy. This is what most American surgeons thought at the time. The University of Maryland Medical Centre reported a series of 175 patients where an intraoperative cholangiogram had been performed. In only 12 (6.8%) patients, filling defects compatible with bile duct stones had been detected and two underwent an ERCP during the same admission and the other 10 were followed up, and of those, only two presented with symptoms requiring ERCP and stone extraction [37]. It therefore transpires that there was a lack of experience and various limitations were acknowledged. This was perhaps due to a lack of laparoscopic instruments and the impression that laparoscopic closure of choledochotomy was a very complex challenge. The manuscript concludes with hope that in the near future new developments will emerge in the laparoscopic management of the ductal stones. When analysing Zucker's work, despite the lack of evidence and experience, they nevertheless were able to support the transcystic approach as, quite rightly, the safest route to accessing the bile duct. Furthermore, they described the use of a choledochoscope with a working channel, which could be railroaded over a guidewire, and then passage of a Dormia basket through the working channel. As a result, 30 years ago they were setting the foundations to develop laparoscopic bile duct exploration. As predicted, the laparoscopic approach to the bile duct was a subject of great interest and research. In the same year Zucker's book was published, Joseph Petelin (Kansas City, USA) published his early experience with laparoscopic biliary ductal evaluation, choledochoscopy and removal of common duct stones in *Surgical Laparoscopy & Endoscopy* [38]. Also in the same year, Moises Jacobs and colleagues (Miami, Florida, USA) described a technique of laparoscopic choledochotomy and placement of a T-tube [39] whereas Sackier, Berci and Paz-Partlow (Los Angeles, California, USA) reported their method for laparoscopic transcystic choledocholithotomy with removal of common duct stones through the cystic duct using a flexible nephroureteroscope [40]. It was just a year later, in 1992, when the first description of lithotripsy during laparoscopic common bile duct exploration (which we refer to as lithotripsy-assisted bile duct exploration by laparoendoscopy or LABEL) was reported by Maurice Arregui et al. (Indianapolis, USA) [41]. The authors described two patients who initially failed preoperative ERCP due to large and/or impacted CBD stones, who were successfully managed by laparoscopic transcystic common bile duct exploration with electrohydraulic lithotripsy. The very same manuscript also reports on 10 patients who underwent laparoscopic cholecystectomy with intraoperative ERCP. Fittingly, some 10 years later, Maurice Arregui wrote about Zucker in a 'Tribute to Karl Zucker: an ambitious, dedicated, and unselfish surgeon of his time' which was published in *Surgical Laparoscopy, Endoscopy and Percutaneous Techniques* [42].

The several millennia of human focus on the gallbladder has seen multiple re-considerations of the role of this organ on health and disease. The early nineteenth century led to understanding that it could be safely removed, and the past 30 years have led to a revolution in minimally invasive approaches that have offered new approaches in the laparoscopic management of biliary disease. The current standard of excellence and future developments, which have been expanded upon in the remainder of this book, will allow improved patient outcomes and patient related outcome measures so that the scourge of biliary disease will be further minimised in years to come.

References

1. Ashrafian H. Avicenna (980-1037) and the first description of post-hepatic jaundice secondary to biliary obstruction. Liver Int. 2014;34(3):479–80.
2. Ashrafian H. Leonardo da Vinci and a cystohepatic triangle anomaly 383 years before Calot. Dig Liver Dis 2013;45(Oct):867–8.
3. Langenbuch C. Ein Fall von Extirpation der Gallenblase wegen chronischer Cholelithiasis. Heilung Berl Klin Wochenschr. 19:725–7.
4. Schupel O. Handbuch der specie lien Pathologie und Theraple. 1883rd ed. Von Ziemsen H, editor. Leipzig; 1883;212:1874–83.
5. Tait L. Cholecystotomy and cholecystectomy. Med News 1884;687–688.
6. Musser JH, Keeu WW. Cholecystotomy with a report of two new cases, a table of all the hitherto reported cases, and remarks. Am J Med Sci. 1884;88:333–67.

7. Jr SH. Justus Ohage-America's premier cholecystectomy surgeon. Missouri Med. 9:86–91.

8. Mayo W. Some observations on the surgery of the gallbladder and the bile-ducts. Ann Surg. 1899;30:452–8.

9. Mayo W. A short discouyrse on surgery of the gallbladder. Surg Gynecol Obs. 1926;43:46–9.

10. Newhook T, Yeo C, Pinckney J, Maxwell IV. John Blair Deaver MD and his Marvelous retractor. Am Surg. 2012;Feb;78:155–6.

11. Soper N. Cholecystectomy: from langenbuch to natural orifice transluminal endoscopic surgery. World J Surg. 2011;35(7):1422–7.

12. Thornton JK. Observations on cases illustrating hepatic surgery.In:proceedings of the medical society in London. Lancet 1891;1:547.

13. Obituary. John Knowsley Thornton MB,Edin CM, JP. Br Med J 1904;Jan 9(1(2245)):109–10.

14. Quintero GA. Cirugía hepatobiliar: Historia y perspectiva. Rev Med 2004;26(67):244–248.

15. Werner OJ, Sohns C, Popov AF, Haskamp J, Schmitto JD. Ludwing Rehn (1849-1930): the German surgeon who performed the worldwide first successful cardiac operation. J Med Biogr. 2012;20(1):2977–82.

16. Jacobson HG, Stern WZ. The Graham-Chole 'test' revisited: the oral cholecystogram today. JAMA. 1883;250(21):2977–82.

17. Reich A. Accidental injection of bile ducts with petrolatum and bismuth paste. JAMA 1918;71(19):1555.

18. Mirizzi P. Operative cholangiography its contribution to the physio-pathology of the common bile duct. Lancet. 1938;232(5998):366–9.

19. Patel JC, Patel J. Cirugia de la via biliar principal. In: Patel JC, Patel J, editors. Tratado de Tecnica Quirurgica XII-2. 2nd ed. Barcelona: Masson; 1980. p. 89–152.

20. Longland CJ. Choledochoscopy in choledocholithiasis. Br J Surg. 1973;60(8):626–8.

21. McCune W, Shorb PE, Moscovitz H. Endoscopic cannulation of the ampulla of Vater. Ann Surg 1968;May:753–5.

22. Ravinov K, Simon M. Peroral cannulation of ampulla of Vater for direct cholangiography and Pancreatography. Radiology. 1965;85:693.

23. Cotton P. Cannulation of the papilla of Vater by endoscopic and retrograde cholangiopancreatography (ERCP). Gut. 1972;13:1014–25.

24. Cotton P, Kruse A. 40 Years of interventional ERCP: stories from the pioneers volume 1 of 2. Channel Cook News Publ. 2014;1(3)

25. Kawai K, Nakajima M, Kimoto K, Sugawara K, Fukumoto K. Endoscopic Sphincterotomy of the Ampulla of Vater. Endoscopy [Internet]. 1975;7(1):30–5. Available from:. https://doi.org/10.1016/S0016-5107(74)73914-1.

26. Classen M, Demling L. Endoskopische Sphinkterotomie der papilla Vateri und Steinextraktion aus dem Ductus choledochus. Dtsch Med Wochenschr. 1974;99(11):496–7.

27. Cholecystectomy HJ. In: Blumgart LH, editor. Surgery of the liver and biliary tract. 1st ed. Edinburgh: Churchill Livingstone; 1988. p. 559–67.

28. Girard RM, Jegros GS. Stones in the common bile duct surgical approaches. In: Blumgart LH, editor. Surgery of the liver and biliary tract. 1st ed. Edinburgh; 1988. p. 577–85.

29. Ashby BS. Operative choledochoscopy in common bile duct surgery. Ann R Coll Surg Engl. 1985;67:279–83.

30. Reynolds W. The first laparoscopic cholecystectomy. JSLS. 2001;5(1):89–94.

31. Litynski GS. Highlights in the history of laparoscopy. In: Litynski GS, editor. Highlights in the history of laparoscopy. Frankfurt: Barbara Bernert Verlag; 1996. p. 131–44.

32. Mühe E. Long-term follow-up after laparoscopic cholecystectomy. Endoscopy. 1992;24:754–8.

33. Litinsky G. Mouret, Dubois, and Perissat: the Laparoscopic breakthrough in Europe. JSLS. 1999;3(2):163–7.

34. Dubois F, Icard P, Berthelot G, Levard H. Coelioscopic Cholecystetomy. Preliminary Report of 36 cases. Ann Surg. 1990;211(1):60–2.

35. Perisat J, Collet D, Belliard R. Gallstones: laparoscopic treatment-cholecystectomy, cholecystostomy and lithotripsy. Surg Endosc 1990;4(1):1–5.

36. Zucker K. Laparoscopic guided cholecystectomy with electro-cautery dissection. In: Zucker K, editor. Surgical laparoscopy. St. Louis Missouri: Quality Medical Publishing Inc; 1991. p. 154.

37. Bailey RW, Zucker KA. Laparoscopic cholangiography and management of Choledocholithiasis. In: Zucker KA, editor. Surgical laparoscopy. St. Louis Missouri: Quality Medical Publishing Inc; 1991. p. 201–25.

38. Petelin J. Laparoscopic approach to common duct pathology. Surg Laparosc Endosc. 1991;1(1):33–41.

39. Jacobs M, Verdeja JC, Goldstein H. Laparoscopic choledocholi-thotomy. J Laparoendosc Adv Surg Tech. 1991;28:79–82.
40. Sackier J, Berci G, Paz-Partlow M. Laparoscopic transcystic choledocholothotomy as an adjunct to laparoscopic cgolecystec-tomy. Am Surg. 1991;57(5):323–6.
41. Arregi M, Davis C, Arkush A, Nagan R. Laparoscopic cholecys-tectomy combined with endoscopic sphincterotomy and stone extraction or laparoscopic choledochoscopy and electrohydrau-lic lithotripsy for management of cholelithiasis with choledocho-lithiasis. Surg Endosc. 1992;6(1):1–15.
42. Arregui M, Scott-Conner C. Tribute to Karl Zucker: an ambi-tious, dedicated, and unselfish surgeon of his time. Surg Laparosc Endosc Percutan Tech 2002;12(3):145–203.

Chapter 2
Review of the Evidence for Laparoscopic Bile Duct Exploration (LBDE)

Lalin Navaratne and Alberto Martinez-Isla

Introduction

Currently, there is no consensus for the optimal treatment of common bile duct (CBD) stones with gallbladder in situ. Guidelines from the British Society of Gastroenterology (BSG) do not report a superiority in efficacy, morbidity or mortality, between laparoscopic cholecystectomy with intra-operative cholangiogram (LC-IOC) ± laparoscopic bile duct exploration (LBDE) and preoperative or intraoperative endoscopic retrograde cholangiopancreatography (ERCP) followed by LC [1]. NICE guidelines recommend the single-stage management LC-IOC ± LBDE, but only provided that the necessary expertise is available [2]. There are 4 strategies available for the management of CBD stones with gallbladder in situ: pre-operative ERCP + LC; LC + LBDE;

L. Navaratne (✉) · A. Martinez-Isla
Northwick Park and St Mark's Hospitals, London North West University Healthcare NHS Trust, London, UK
e-mail: lalin.navaratne@doctors.org.uk; a.isla@imperial.ac.uk

A. Martinez-Isla, L. Navaratne (eds.), *Laparoscopic Common Bile Duct Exploration*, In Clinical Practice,
https://doi.org/10.1007/978-3-030-93203-9_2

LC + intra-operative ERCP and finally LC + post-operative ERCP. Multiple randomised control trials (RCT) have been performed in the last 20 years comparing these 4 treatments followed by numerous systematic reviews in the last 10 years (Tables 2.1, 2.2 and 2.3) trying to identify the best management strategy for choledocholithiasis with concomitant gallstones [3–14].

TABLE 2.1 Systematic reviews of the management of choledocholithiasis within the last 10 years

Author Year	Management of concomitant gallstones and CBD stones	No. of RCTs (patients)
Li 2011	LC + LCBDE vs pre-op ERCP+ LC	5 RCT (621)
	LC + LCBDE vs LC + post-op ERCP	2 RCT (166)
	Pre-op ERCP vs LC + intra-op ERCP	3 RCT (412)
	Pre-op ERCP + LC vs LC + post-op ERCP	1 RCT (59)
Alexakis 2012	One-stage laparoendoscopic (LC + LCBDE and LC + intra-op ERCP) vs two-stage (pre-op ERCP + LC and LC + post-op ERCP)	9 RCT (933)
Lu 2012	One-stage (LC + LCBDE) vs two-stage (pre-op ERCP+ LC and LC + post-op ERCP)	7 RCT (787)
Dasari 2013	LC + LCBDE vs pre-op ERCP+ LC	5 RCT (621)
	LC + LCBDE vs LC + intra-op ERCP	1 RCT (234)
	LC + LCBDE vs LC + post-op ERCP	2 RCT (166)
	One-stage vs two-stage	7 RCT (787)

TABLE 2.1 (continued)

Author Year	Management of concomitant gallstones and CBD stones	No. of RCTs (patients)
Liu 2014	LC + LCBDE vs LC + EST (studies include pre-op, intra-op and post-op ERCP)	15 RCT (1410)
Nagaraja 2014	LC + LCBDE vs pre-op ERCP + LC	6 RCT (741)
	LC + LCBDE vs LC + post-op ERCP	2 RCT (166)
	LC + LCBDE vs LC + intra-op ERCP	2 RCT (453)
	Pre-op ERCP + LC vs LC + intra-op ERCP	5 RCT (632)
Zhu 2015	One-stage (LC + LCBDE) vs two-stage (pre-op ERCP + LC)	8 RCT (1130)
Prasson 2016	One-stage laparoendoscopic (LC + LCBDE and LC + intra-op ERCP) vs two-stage (pre-op ERCP + LC and LC + post-op ERCP)	14 RCT (1600)
Gao 2017	LC + LCBDE vs LC + EST (studies include pre-op, intra-op and post-op ERCP)	11 RCT (1663)
Ricci 2018	LCBDE	20 RCT (2489)
	Pre-op ERCP + LC	
	LC + post-op ERCP	
	LC + intra-op ERCP	
Singh 2018	One-stage (LC + LCBDE) vs two-stage (pre-op ERCP + LC)	11 RCT (1513)
Li 2019	One-stage (LC + LCBDE) vs two-stage (pre-op ERCP + LC and LC + post-op ERCP)	11 RCT (1338)

TABLE 2.2 Systematic reviews of the management of choledocholithiasis within the last 10 years

Author Year	Stone clearance	Morbidity (%)	Mortality (%)	Hospital stay	Cost
Li 2011	↑LCBDE (1 RCT)	No difference	No difference	↓LCBDE (2 RCT)	Not extractable
	No difference	No difference	No difference	↓LCBDE (1 RCT)	Not extractable
	No difference	↓intra-op ERCP (1 RCT)	No difference	↓intra-op ERCP (3 RCT)	↓intra-op ERCP (2 RCT)
	No difference	No difference	No difference	↓post-op ERCP (1 RCT)	↓post-op ERCP (1 RCT)
Alexakis 2012	No difference	No difference 19.9% vs 16.1% (p = 0.10)	No difference	Not reported	↓one-stage laparoendoscopic (2 RCT)
Lu 2012	No difference 87.2% vs 78.8% (p = 0.17)	No difference 19.0% vs 15.2% (p = 0.16)	No difference	No difference	↓one-stage (1 RCT)

	↑LCBDE (1 RCT)	No difference	No difference	↓LCBDE (2 RCT)	↓one-stage (1 RCT)
Dasari 2013	↑LCBDE (1 RCT)	No difference	No difference	↓LCBDE (2 RCT)	↓one-stage (1 RCT)
	No difference	No difference	No difference	No difference	No difference
	↑LCBDE (p < 0.05)[a]	No difference	No difference	↓LCBDE (1 RCT)	Not extractable
	↑LCBDE (p = 0.03)[a]	No difference	No difference	Not reported	Not extractable
Liu 2014	92.7% vs 89.1% (OR 1.55, p = 0.03)	No difference	Not reported	↓LCBDE WMD − 3.32d (p < 0.05)	↓LC + LCBDE (4 RCT)
Nagaraja 2014	No difference	No difference	No difference	No difference	Not extractable
	No difference	No difference	Not reported	3.7d v 5.6d (p = 0.19)	Not extractable
	No difference	No difference	No difference	No difference	Not extractable
	No difference	No difference	No difference	6.1d v 3.5d (p < 0.01)	No difference

(continued)

TABLE 2.2 (continued)

Author Year	Stone clearance	Morbidity (%)	Mortality (%)	Hospital stay	Cost
Zhu 2015	90.2% vs 85.7% (OR 1.56, p = 0.03)	No difference	No difference	↓one-stage WMD − 1.02d (p = 0.04)	Not extractable
Prasson 2016	82.0% vs 78.8% (p = 0.15)	No difference	No difference	No difference WMD 1.31d (p = 0.17)	Not extractable
Gao 2017	No difference	No difference	No difference	No difference	Not extractable
Ricci 2018	Sucra 55.7% Mean rank 2	Sucra 43.9% Mean rank 3	Sucra 54.1% Mean rank 2	Sucra 68.0% Mean rank 2	Sucra 98.9% Mean rank 1
	Sucra 44.3% Mean rank 3	Sucra 23.8% Mean rank 4	Sucra 53.8% Mean rank 2	Sucra 22.1% Mean rank 3	Sucra 11.5% Mean rank 3
	Sucra 12.8% Mean rank 4	Sucra 62.7% Mean rank 2	Sucra 53.9% Mean rank 2	Sucra 17.2% Mean rank 4	Not reported
	Sucra 87.2% Mean rank 1	Sucra 69.7% Mean rank 2	Sucra 38.2% Mean rank 3	Sucra 92.7% Mean rank 1	Sucra 39.6% Mean rank 2

Singh 2018	↑one-stage OR 0.59 (p = 0.02)[b]	No difference	No difference	↓one-stage WMD – 1.63d (p = 0.05)	↓one-stage (2 RCT)
Li 2019	No difference	No difference	No difference	No difference	Not extractable

WMD weighted mean difference, *SUCRA* surface under the cumulative ranking curve

[a]On fixed-effect analysis

[b]Rate of technical failure

TABLE 2.3 Randomised studies included in the systematic reviews of the management of choledocholithiasis within the last 10 years

Trial	Author	Li 2011	Alexakis 2012	Lu 2012	Dasari 2013	Liu 2014	Nagaraja 2014	Zhu 2015	Prasson 2016	Gao 2017	Ricci 2018	Singh 2018	Li 2019
A	Cuschieri	X	X	X	X	X	X	X	X	X	X	X	X
	Sgourakis	X	X	X	X	X	X	X	X	X	X	X	X
	Pi[a]					X							
	Chen[a]					X							
	Noble	X	X	X	X	X	X	X	X	X	X	X	X
	Rogers	X	X	X	X	X	X	X	X	X	X	X	X
	Bansal	X	X	X	X	X	X	X	X	X	X	X	X
	Dai[a]					X							
	Li[a]					X							
	Liao[a]					X							
	Ferulano								X		X	X	
	Li[a]					X							
	Shen[a]					X							
	Koc						X	X	X	X	X	X	X
	Ding							X	X		X	X	X
	Bansal							X	X	X		X	X
	Lv										X	X	X
	Gonzalez											X	X

B	Rhodes	X	X		X		X	X		X			X		X
	Nathanson	X	X		X		X	X		X			X	X	X
C	Hong				X		X		X	X					X
	ElGeidie						X	X		X		X		X	X
	Poh											X		X	X
D	Lella	X					X		X					X	X
	Rabago	X					X		X					X	X
	Morino	X	X				X		X	X			X	X	X
	ElGeidie	X					X		X					X	X
	Tzovaras		X				X		X	X			X	X	X
E	Sahoo									X			X	X	X
	Chang[a]	X								X			X	X	X

A, LC + LCBDE vs pre-op ERCP + LC. B, LC + LCBDE vs LC + post-op ERCP. C, LC + LCBDE vs LC + intra-op ERCP. D, Pre-op ERCP vs LC + intra-op ERCP. E, Pre-op ERCP + LC vs LC + post-op ERCP

[a] Article in Chinese

Stone Clearance

Zhu et al., and Singh et al., compared LC + LCBDE *vs* two-stage (preoperative ERCP + LC) and found LC ± LBDE achieved significantly higher stone clearance rates (Table 2.2). Zhu et al., included 1130 patients from 8 RCTs and found clearance rates of 90.2% *vs* 85.7% (OR 1.56; 95% Confidence Interval 1.05 to 2.33, p = 0.03) in favour of LC + LBDE [10]. Singh et al., studied 1513 patients from 11 RCTs and reported higher rates of stone clearance from patients receiving LC + LBDE (92.7% vs 89.1%; OR 1.55, p = 0.03) [13]. Liu et al. compared laparoscopic *vs* endoscopic management of CBD stones and found higher stone clearance rates with laparoscopic techniques (92.7% vs 89.1%; OR 1.55, p = 0.03) [8]. Two further systematic reviews of RCTs found superior LC + LBDE clearance rates but these did not reach statistical significance (87.2% vs 78.8%, p = 0.17 and 82.0% vs 78.8%, p = 0.15 [6, 11]. Ricci et al., performed a network meta-analysis of RCTs and reported that LC + intraoperative ERCP was the approach with the greatest probability of success (surface under the cumulative ranking curve (SUCRA) 87.2%), followed by LC + LBDE (SUCRA 55.7%), preoperative ERCP + LC (SUCRA 44.3%) and finally LC + postoperative ERCP (SUCRA 12.8%) [12].

Morbidity

Alexakis et al., conducted a systematic review of one-stage laparoendoscopic (LC-IOC + LBDE and LC + intraoperative ERCP) versus two-stage management of CBD stones (preoperative ERCP + LC and LC + postoperative ERCP) and the authors found a non-significant trend towards increased morbidity within the one-stage group (19.9% vs 16.1%, p = 0.10) [5]. This was consistent with Lu et al. findings, who also described a trend towards increased morbidity within the one-stage group (19.0% *vs* 15.2%, p = 0.16) [6]. Liu et al., included 15 RCTs and 1410 patients in their comparison of laparoscopic versus endoscopic (including pre-, intra- and postoperative ERCP) management of ductal stones and did not find any difference between the groups in terms of overall morbidity (15.4% *vs* 18.8%, p = 0.58), however, reported a higher bile leak rate within the laparoscopic group (6.3% vs 0.5%) and a higher incidence of bleeding and pancreatitis in the endoscopic group (0% *vs* 3.7% and 0.3% *vs* 3.6% respectively) [8]. Rabago et al., randomised patients with choledocholithiasis to either preoperative ERCP + LC or LC + intraoperative ERCP, and reported favourable morbidity outcomes in the latter single-stage group (23% vs 8.5%, p < 0.05) [15]. Ricci et al., in terms of morbidity, found LC + intraoperative ERCP to be the safest approach (SUCRA 69.7%), followed by LC + postoperative ERCP, LC-IOC ± LBDE, and finally preoperative ERCP + LC (SUCRA 62.7%, 43.9%, 23.8% respectively) [12].

Bile Leak

As discussed, LC-IOC ± LBDE appears to be neither superior nor inferior to endoscopic techniques in terms of overall morbidity for treating bile duct stones, however its morbidity, is mainly represented by bile leak. Ricci et al., included in their meta-analysis 915 patients from 14 RCTs that underwent LC + LBDE (Table 2.3), but from these trials, only 331 (36.2%) patients had their duct explored via the transcystic route [12]. Furthermore, during the last two decades, 23 RCTs have compared LC + LBDE with other therapeutic options, and from 16 studies published in English, the transcystic approach was used in just 32% (305/953) of patients (Table 2.4). In five trials, the sole method of LBDE was via choledochotomy (transductal approach) [16–20]. When the transcystic route was attempted, the success rate for stone clearance was 80% (from extractable data). A recent review in 2020 found that the transcystic approach can be achieved in up to 71% of cases [21], however, higher transcystic rates approaching 90% have been reported [22, 23]. Series with

TABLE 2.4 Attempted and success rates of transcystic LCBDE with surgeon's experience in LCBDE from 16 RCTs performed within last 20 years

Paper	Year	Attempted Transcystic LCBDE (%)	Transcystic success rate (%)	LCBDE surgeon experience
Cuschieri	1999	56/111 (50.5)	45/56 (80.4)	Varying experience NOS
Sgourakis	2002	20/35 (57.1)	Not extractable	Not extractable
Noble	2009	5/44 (11.4)	5/5 (100)	Experienced biliary surgeons/ trainees under supervision
Rogers	2010	17/17 (100)	15/17 (88.2)	Single surgeon with extensive experience
Bansal	2010	0/15 (0)	N/A	Early institutional experience
Ferulano	2011	55/62 (88.7)	29/38 (76.3)	Not extractable
Koc	2013	0/57 (0)	N/A	Two experienced hepatobiliary surgeons
Ding	2014	0/110 (0)	N/A	Single surgeon with extensive experience
Bansal	2014	1/84 (1.2)	1/1 (100)	Early institutional experience

TABLE 2.4 (continued)

Paper	Year	Attempted Transcystic LCBDE (%)	Transcystic success rate (%)	LCBDE surgeon experience
Lv	2016	23/29 **(79.3)**	23/23 **(100)**	Not extractable
Gonzalez	2016	Not extractable	Not extractable	Three experienced laparoscopic surgeons
Rhodes	1998	28/40 **(70)**	23/28 **(82.1)**	29/40 by consultant (experience unknown). 11/40 by trainee
Nathanson	2005	0/41 **(0)**	N/A	Experienced laparoscopic surgeons
Hong	2006	0/141 **(0)**	N/A	Not extractable
ElGeidie	2011	57/115 **(49.6)**	Not extractable	Not extractable
Poh	2016	43/52 **(82.7)**	29/43 **(67.4)**	Individual experience of 10–40 cases
Total		305/953 **(32.0)**	170/211 **(80.6)**	

high rates of transductal exploration have reported bile leak rates as high as 13.3–16.7% [16, 24]. Therefore, the advantages of easier access and extraction of stones from the transductal (transcholedochal) approach are taxed with complications, mainly in the form of bile leak. In series with high rates of transductal exploration, bile leakage will highlight the main weakness of the LC-IOC ± LBDE approach when compared to the other endoscopic techniques. Liu et al., reported that the total incidences of bile leakage in the laparoscopic and endoscopic groups from eight studies included in their systematic review were 6.3% and 0.5% respectively [8]. Reinders et al., published a systematic review on transcystic versus transductal stone extraction during single-stage treatment of choledochocystolithiasis in 2014 [25]. Expectedly, the authors found that there were more bile leaks after transductal stone extraction (11% vs 1.7%, p < 0.5) and total morbidity was also significantly less in the transcystic group (7–10.5% vs 18.4–26.7%, p < 0.05). Pang et al., more recently published their results from a similar study and found that transcystic exploration had significantly shorter operative time and hospital stay, less operative blood loss, fewer complications and was more cost efficient than traditional transductal LBDE [26]. From the authors institution and review of over four hundred LBDEs, the rate of bile leak from transductal and transcystic exploration was 5.8% and 1.1% respectively (p = 0.02) [23]. Furthermore, Ricci and colleagues found that regarding biliary leak, the worst approach was 'undoubtedly' LBDE when compared to pre-, intra- or postoperative ERCP with laparoscopic cholecystectomy [12]. However, when approximately only a third of patients included in their systematic review (and all RCTs conducted within the last two decades) received transcystic LBDE, it is perhaps likely that the overall reported morbidity associated with bile leak from the LBDE arm overrepresents the true morbidity associated with a contemporary transcystic predominant LBDE practice.

Post-Procedural Pancreatitis

The rate of post-procedure pancreatitis has been reported as being higher in endoscopic groups (pre-, intra- or postoperative ERCP with LC) when compared to LC + LBDE groups [8, 12]. This difference is still apparent despite many of the randomised trials having included a substantial proportion of patients within the LC + LBDE arm who underwent closure of choledochotomy over an antegrade stent [19, 27–29]. It is known that this technique appears to be associated with pancreatitis due to instrumentation of the biliary sphincter [30]. The incidence of pancreatitis following closure over an antegrade stent has been reported to be as high as 12% with 26% of patients becoming hyperamylasaemic [23, 31]. At the authors institution, if it is not possible to explore the bile duct through the transcystic approach and the transductal route is used, the duct is currently closed primarily without an antegrade stent [23]. As with morbidity secondary to bile leak, it is likely that if individual randomised studies had higher rates of transcystic stone extraction, the overall morbidity associated with LBDE (in terms of bile leak and pancreatitis) would be lower than that currently reported in the systematic reviews. Future research consisting of large, multicentre prospective studies with strict trial protocols for transcystic exploration (where possible) are required to identify morbidity associated with a contemporary transcystic predominant LBDE practice.

Hospital Stay and Cost

There is fairly robust evidence to support shorter hospital stay in LC + LBDE groups when compared to endoscopic (pre-, intra- and postoperative ERCP) groups [8] and two-stage (preoperative ERCP + LC) groups [10, 13]. Nagaraja et al., studied 632 patients from 5 RCTs of preoperative ERCP + LC versus LC + intraoperative ERCP and found shorter hospital stay within the latter group (6.1 *vs* 3.5 days, p < 0.01) [9]. However, the authors did not find any differences in length of hospital stay when comparing LC + LBDE to pre-, intra- or postoperative ERCP [9]. Furthermore, Ricci and co-workers found that the shortest hospital stay was when LC + intraoperative ERCP was performed (SUCRA 92.7%), followed by LC + LBDE (SUCRA 68.0%), preoperative ERCP + LC (SUCRA 22.1%) and LC + postoperative ERCP (SUCRA 17.2%) [12]. Two RCTs comparing LC + LCBDE vs preoperative ERCP + LC and one RCT comparing LC + LBDE vs LC + postoperative ERCP have demonstrated shorter hospital stay with LCBDE [16, 27, 28]. Chang et al., randomised patients with gallstones pancreatitis to preoperative ERCP + LC or LC-IOC with selective postoperative ERCP in patients with a positive IOC, and reported reduced cost and hospital stay in the selective postoperative ERCP group [32]. However, according to most guidelines, the common bile duct should be cleaned before or during laparoscopic cholecystectomy [2, 33–35]. The remainder of the systematic reviews listed in Tables 2.1 and 2.2 did not find any difference in length of hospital stay between treatment groups [3–6, 11].

Two randomised studies comparing preoperative ERCP + LC with LC + intraoperative ERCP have demonstrated significantly less cost associated with the single-stage procedure [15, 36]. Another randomised study comparing LC + LBDE with preoperative ERCP + LC reported reduced costs with the single-stage group [16]. Ricci et al., considered total cost in US dollars of the four different treatment strategies and concluded that the procedure with the highest probability of being the least expensive was LC + LBDE (SUCRA 98.9%), followed by LC + intraoperative ERCP (SUCRA 39.6%) and preoperative ERCP + LC (SUCRA 11.5%) [12].

Learning Curve and Teaching

The first published reports of LBDE came from the early 1990s with data extracted from randomised studies discussed in this chapter from 1998 onwards. This year also coincides with the same year the technique was started in the authors institution [23]. Published reports for ERCP date back to the mid-1970s, however, the earliest study of intraoperative ERCP included in systematic reviews was 2006. With the two techniques sitting apart on the learning curve, ERCP has had a two-decade head start when compared to LCBDE. The learning curve of LBDE has been demonstrated at the authors institution which spans 20 years. The success rate of stone clearance in chronological blocks of 100 cases has, as expected, increased with experience: 90%, 98%, 97%, 100% and increasing use of transcystic choledochoscopy has also been observed. Lessons learned after the first 200 LBDE cases was published in 2014, and at that time, the transductal exploration rate was 88.5% [31]. At the beginning of the series, closure of the duct over a T-tube was performed but subsequently closure over an antegrade stent was preferred. However, due to a high incidence of acute pancreatitis, primary closure was then adopted. At that time, primary closure of the duct after LBDE seemed to be superior to closure over a T tube and stent, but this was a lesson learned only after almost 200 cases. The complication rate of pancreatitis was 6.8% in the first half of the series (~200 cases) which has reduced to less than 1% in the latter half of the series (~200 cases).

It is important to consider technical experience prior to drawing any firm conclusions from a study (Table 2.4). Poh et al., published a study comparing LC + intraoperative ERCP with LBDE, and operator experience of LCBDE was comparatively lower than that of ERCP being between 10 and 40 cases only [29]. Within the UK, ERCP endoscopists must achieve a benchmark of 180 cases in training with a minimum of 75 cases per year to retain their competency [37]. For LBDE, 250 cases has been described as the learning curve for competency by some authors [38]. Within the UK, there is a standardised ERCP training pathway delivered by the Joint Advisory Group (JAG) on GI Endoscopy and almost every hospital has a gastroenterology department offering an ERCP service. Conversely, there are just a few hospitals offering a LC-IOC ± LBDE service with audited outcomes and reliable clinical pathways. Table 2.4 shows the operator experience of the surgeons who participated in each of the 16 RCTs published in English within the last 20 years.

Two studies reported a proportion of the operations being performed by trainee surgeons [28, 39]. Another study was performed in a centre with very early institutional experience of LBDE [16]. In a large multicentre trial administered through the European Association of Endoscopic Surgeons (EAES), participating surgeons from several European centres and Australia had varying experience in LBDE at the beginning of the trial [27]. The investigators described this as the main strength of the study stating that it was pragmatic and therefore the results were applicable generally, not just in centres with specialised expertise in laparoscopic biliary surgery. We believe that LBDE should be considered specialist practice and therefore only performed by surgeons who have had specific training in LCBDE and advanced laparoscopic techniques [40]. In accordance with UK NICE guidelines, we recommend that LBDE should be offered in all centres receiving emergency surgical patients and performed by surgeons with regular exposure to managing CBD stones [2]. We advocate that LCBDE should be included as part of the mandatory training for upper gastrointestinal surgeons (see Chapter on mentoring and training).

References

1. Williams E, Beckingham I, El Sayed G, et al. Updated guideline on the management of common bile duct stones (CBDS). Gut. 2017;66:765–82.
2. NICE Clinical Guideline. Gallstones disease: Diagnosis and management. 2014.
3. Gao YC, Chen J, Qin Q, Chen H, Wang W, Zhao J, et al. Efficacy and safety of laparoscopic bile duct exploration versus endoscopic sphincterotomy for concomitant gallstones and common bile duct stones. Medicine (United States). 2017;96(37):e7925.
4. Li Z-Q, Sun J-X, Li B, Dai X-Q, Yu A-X, Li Z-F. Meta-analysis of single-stage versus two-staged management for concomitant gallstones and common bile duct stones. J Minim Access Surg. 2020;16(3):206–14. https://doi.org/10.4103/JMAS_146_18.

5. Alexakis N, Connor S. Meta-analysis of one- vs. two-stage laparoscopic/endoscopic management of common bile duct stones. HPB. 2012;14(4):254–9.

6. Lu J, Cheng Y, Xiong XZ, Lin YX, Wu SJ, Cheng NS. Two-stage vs single-stage management for concomitant gallstones and common bile duct stones. World J Gastroenterol. 2012;18(24):3156–66.

7. Dasari B, Tan C, Gurusamy KS, Martin D, Kirk G, Mckie L, et al. Surgical versus endoscopic treatment of bile duct stones (review) summary of findings for the main comparison. Cochrane Database Syst Rev 2013;12.

8. Liu J, Wang Y, Shu G, Lou C, Zhang J, Du Z. Laparoscopic versus endoscopic Management of Choledocholithiasis in patients undergoing laparoscopic cholecystectomy: a meta-analysis. J Laparoendosc Adv Surg Tech [Internet]. 2014;24(5):287–94. Available from: http://online.liebertpub.com/doi/abs/10.1089/lap.2013.0546

9. Nagaraja V, Eslick G, Cox M. Systematic review and meta-analysis of minimally invasive techniques for the management of cholecysto-choledocholithiasis. J Hepatobiliary Pancreat Sci. 2014;21(12):896–901.

10. Zhu H, Xu M, Shen H, Yang C, Li F, Li K, et al. A meta-analysis of single-stage versus two-stage management for concomitant gallstones and common bile duct stones. Clin Res Hepatol Gastroenterol. 2015;39(5):584–93.

11. Prasson P, Bai X, Zhang Q, Liang T. One-stage laproendoscopic procedure versus two-stage procedure in the management for gallstone disease and biliary duct calculi: a systemic review and meta-analysis. Surg Endosc. 2016;30(8):3582–90.

12. Ricci C, Pagano N, Taffurelli G, Pacilio C, Migliori M, Bazzoli F, et al. Comparison of efficacy and safety of 4 combinations of laparoscopic and intraoperative techniques for management of gallstone disease with Biliary Duct Calculi. JAMA Surg [Internet]. 2018:e181167. Available from: http://archsurg.jamanetwork.com/article.aspx?doi=10.1001/jamasurg.2018.1167

13. Singh A, Kilambi R. Single-stage laparoscopic common bile duct exploration and cholecystectomy versus two-stage endoscopic stone extraction followed by laparoscopic cholecystectomy for patients with gallbladder stones with common bile duct stones: systematic review and meta. Surg Endosc [Internet]. 2018;32(9):3763–3776. Available from: https://doi.org/10.1007/s00464-018-6170-8.

14. Li MK, Tang CN, Lai EC. Managing concomitant gallbladder stones and common bile duct stones in the laparoscopic era: a systematic review. Asian J Endosc Surg. 2011;4(2):53–8.

15. Rabago LR, Vicente C, Solar F, et al. Two-stage treatment with preoperative endoscopic retrograde cholangiopancreatogtaphy (ERCP) compared with single stage treatment with intraoperative ERCP for patients with symptomatic cholelithiasis with possible choledocholithiasis. Endoscopy. 2006;30:779–86.

16. Rogers SJ, Cello JP, Horn JK, Siperstein AE, Schecter WP, Campbell AR, et al. Prospective randomized trial of LC+LCBDE vs ERCP/S+LC for common bile duct stone disease. Arch Surg. 2010;145(1):28–33.

17. Koc B, Karahan S, Adas G, Tutal F, Guven H, Ozsoy A. Comparison of laparoscopic common bile duct exploration and endoscopic retrograde cholangiopancreatography plus laparoscopic cholecystectomy for choledocholithiasis: a prospective randomized study. Am J Surg [Internet] 2013;206(4):457–463. Available from: https://doi.org/10.1016/j.amjsurg.2013.02.004.

18. Ding G, Cai W, Qin M, Single-Stage vs. Two-stage management for concomitant gallstones and common bile duct stones: a prospective randomized trial with long-term follow-up. J Gastrointest Surg. 2014;18(5):947–51.

19. Nathanson L, O'Rourke N, Martin I, Fielding G, Cowen A, Roberts R, et al. Postoperative ERCP versus laparoscopic choledochotomy for clearance of selected bile duct calculi: a randomized trial. Ann Surg. 2005;242(2):188–92.

20. Hong DF, Xin Y, Chen DW. Comparison of laparoscopic cholecystectomy combined with intraoperative endoscopic sphincterotomy and laparoscopic exploration of the common bile duct for cholecystocholedocholithiasis. Surg Endosc Other Interv Tech. 2006;20(3):424–7.

21. Narula V, Fung E, Overby D, Richardson W, Stefanidis D. Clinical spotlight review for the management of choledocholithiasis. Surg Endosc [Internet]. 2020;0123456789. Available from: https://doi.org/10.1007/s00464-020-07462-2.

22. Jones T, Al Musawi J, Navaratne L, Martinez-Isla A. Holmium laser lithotripsy improves the rate of successful transcystic laparoscopic common bile duct exploration. Langenbeck's Arch Surg. 2019;404(8):985–92.

23. Navaratne L, Martinez-Isla A. Transductal versus transcystic laparoscopic common bile duct exploration: an institutional review of over four hundred cases. Surg Endosc. 2020;

24. Bansal V, Misra M, Rajan K, Kilambi R, Kumar S, Krishna A, et al. Single-stage laparoscopic common bile duct exploration and cholecystectomy versus two-stage endoscopic stone extraction followed by laparoscopic cholecystectomy for patients with concomitant gallbladder stones and common bile duct stones: a randomized con. Surg Endosc. 2014;28(3):875–85.

25. Reinders JSK, Gouma D, Ubbink DT, Van ramshort B, Boerma D. Transcystic or transductal stone extraction during single stage treatment of choledochocystolithiasis: a systematic review. World J Surg. 2014;38:2403–11.

26. Pang L, Zhang Y, Wang Y, Kong J. Transcystic versus traditional laparoscopic common bile duct exploration: its advantages and a meta-analysis. Surg Endosc. 2018;32:4363–76.

27. Cuschieri A, Lezoche E, Morino M, Croce E, Lacy A, Toouli J, et al. E.A.E.S. multicenter prospective randomized trial comparing two-stage vs single-stage management of patients with gallstone disease and ductal calculi. Surg Endosc. 1999;13(10):952–7.

28. Rhodes M, Sussman L, Cohen LLM. Randomised trial of laparoscopic exploration of common bile duct versus postoperative endoscopic retrograde cholangiography for common bile duct stones. Lancet. 1998;351:159–61.

29. Poh BR, Ho SPS, Sritharan M, Yeong CC, Swan MP, Devonshire DA, et al. Randomized clinical trial of intraoperative endoscopic retrograde cholangiopancreatography versus laparoscopic bile duct exploration in patients with choledocholithiasis. Br J Surg. 2016;103(9):1117–24.

30. Paganini AM, Guerrieri M, Sarnari J, De Sanctis A, D'Ambrosio G, Lezoche G, et al. Thirteen years' experience with laparoscopic transcystic common bile duct exploration for stones. Surg Endosc [Internet] 2007;21(1):34–40. Available from: https://doi.org/10.1007/s00464-005-0286-3.

31. Abellán Morcillo I, Qurashi K, Martinez Isla. A Exploración laparoscópica de la vía biliar, lecciones aprendidas tras más de 200 casos. Cir Esp.2014;92(5):341–47. https://doi.org/10.1016/j.ciresp.2013.02.010.

32. Chang L, Lo S, Stabile BE, Lewis RJ, Toosie K, De Virgilio C. Preoperative versus postoperative endoscopic retrograde cholangiopancreatography in mild to moderate gallstone pancreatitis: a prospective randomized trial. Ann Surg. 2000;231(1):82–7.

33. Sauerland S, Agresta F, Bergamaschi R, Borzellino G, Budzynski A, Champault G, et al. Laparoscopy for abdominal emergencies: evidence-based guidelines of the European Association

for Endoscopic Surgery. Surg Endosc Other Interv Tech. 2006;20(1):14–29.

34. Isaacs P. Endoscopic retrograde cholangiopancreatography training in the United Kingdom: a critical review. World J Gastrointest Endosc 2011;Feb(16)(3(2)):30–3.

35. The Victoria Surgical Consultative Council (VSCC)Guidelines. Complications of ERCP 2007.

36. Morino M, Baracchi F, Miglietta C, Furlan N, Ragona R, Garbarini A. Preoperative endoscopic sphincterotomy versus laparoendoscopic rendezvous in patients with gallbladder and bile duct stones. Ann Surg. 2006;244(6):889–93.

37. ERCP Working Party. BS of G. ERCP – the way forward. A Standards framework 2014.

38. Zhu JG, Han W, Guo W, Su W, Bai ZG, Zhang ZT. Learning curve and outcome of laparoscopic transcystic common bile duct exploration for choledocholithiasis. Br J Surg. 2015;102(13):1691–7.

39. Noble H, Tranter S, Chesworth T, Norton S, Thompson M. A randomized, clinical trial to compare endoscopic Sphincterotomy and subsequent laparoscopic cholecystectomy with primary laparoscopic bile duct exploration during cholecystectomy in higher risk patients with Choledocholithiasis. J Laparoendosc Adv Surg Tech [Internet]. 2009;19(6):713–20. Available from: http://www.liebertonline.com/doi/abs/10.1089/lap.2008.0428

40. Al-Musawi J, Navaratne L, Martinez-Isla A. Laparosocopic common bile ducxt exploration versus endoscopic retrograde cholangiopancreatography for choledocholithiasis found at time of laparoscopic cholecystectomy. Am J Surg. 2018;

Chapter 3
Laparoscopic Biliary Ultrasound

Stuart Andrews and Kirk Bowling

Laparoscopic intra-operative ultrasound (LUS) as a modality for investigating the bile duct in biliary surgery is gaining popularity for a number of reasons. It is rapid, gives accurate and reliable information for treatment and can provide significant advantages in efficiency of patient care.

Evidence shows that LUS is equally as sensitive and specific as MRCP or intra-operative cholangiogram in the detection and exclusion of bile duct stones [1–5]. The process of acquiring images using LUS is significantly quicker than x-ray cholangiogram [6], remains within the surgeon's control and negates the need for potentially dangerous radiation exposure. There is also a growing practice of using intra-operative LUS as an alternative to pre-operative MRCP in those patients who have indices to suggest synchronous common bile duct stones (CBDs) when presenting with symptomatic gallbladder stones. Currently in the UK 1/3 of the 66,000 patients undergoing Laparoscopic Cholecystectomy have a pre-operative MRCP; less than 10% of these patients will have CBDs [7, 8]. LUS can reliably identify and reassure these

S. Andrews (✉) · K. Bowling
South Devon Upper GI Unit, Torbay Hospital, Torquay, UK
e-mail: stuart.n.andrews@nhs.net; kirk.bowling@nhs.net

© The Author(s), under exclusive license to Springer Nature Switzerland AG 2022
A. Martinez-Isla, L. Navaratne (eds.), *Laparoscopic Common Bile Duct Exploration*, In Clinical Practice,
https://doi.org/10.1007/978-3-030-93203-9_3

negative CBDs patients, those patients that have CBDs identified can proceed with treatment either with laparoscopic common bile duct exploration (LCBDE) or post-operative ERCP.

For those surgeons providing a LCBDE service, large amounts of information can be acquired from an LUS other than just exclusion of duct stones. When CBDs are identified, they can be measured in size and number, CBD diameter and cystic duct diameter can be measured, which provides decision making information for LCBDE in terms of trans-cystic vs choledocotomy. LUS naturally compliments a LCBDE service and once experienced it is quickly adopted as a standard of practice.

Equipment

Laparoscopic ultrasound machines are compact and mobile (Fig. 3.1). The probes come in two types, a fixed straight type and flexible type (Fig. 3.2), they most commonly use a linear array transducer and operate at a frequency of 4–10 MHz giving a typical tissue penetration of 3–8 cm, ample for detailed scanning of the porta hepatis and views through the pancreas of the intra-pancreatic portion of the CBD. The flexible type can have more applications for liver/pancreatic imaging, however some surgeons prefer the fixed type probe if to be used exclusively for CBD imaging to allow more controlled handling characteristics, although flexible probes have locking levers which emulates this to some degree. Probes all have common characteristics, they are real-time B-mode, providing high quality images, colour doppler capability is necessary in order to identify and navigate anatomy of the porta. A typical probe has a diameter of 10 mm to allow use down a standard size 11 mm epigastric port used in laparoscopic cholecystectomy, if you are using the American technique or the left upper quadrant port for those using the French technique. The probes are typically 40–50 cm long and can be place alongside other laparoscopic instruments making the LUS set-up very ergonomic and space efficient (Fig. 3.3).

FIGURE 3.1
Laparoscopic ultra-
sound machine

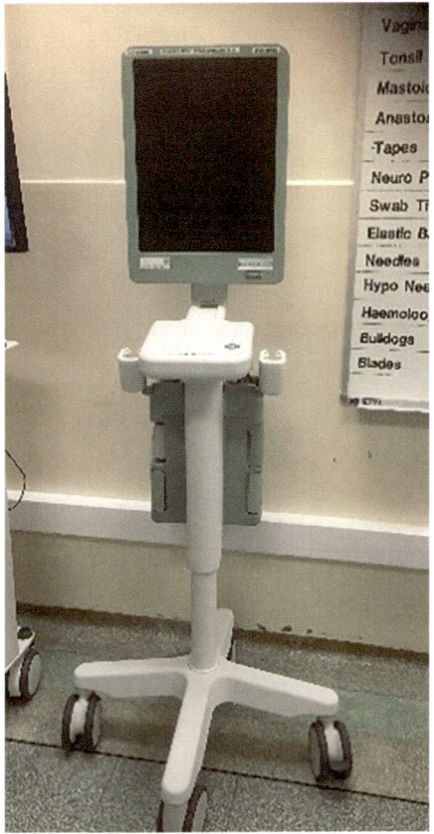

Probe sterility for each patient use can be either with a sheath cover (Fig. 3.4) and probes disinfected between patients, or formally sent away to the hospital sterilisation department between each use (Fig. 3.5). This is an important consideration when purchasing equipment volume, as if a formally sterilisation process is adopted several probes will need to be purchased (at least 5) in order to provide a continuous service for multiple patients on a list and morning/afternoon lists-(approximately 6 h turnaround time). It is important that you agree sterilisation protocols with your infection control department when deciding equipment numbers to purchase in your business case.

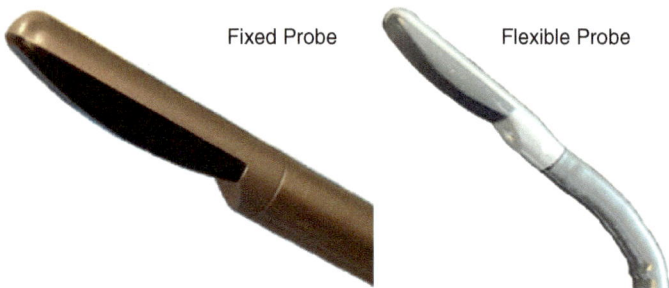

Fixed Probe   Flexible Probe

FIGURE 3.2 Laparoscopic ultrasound probes

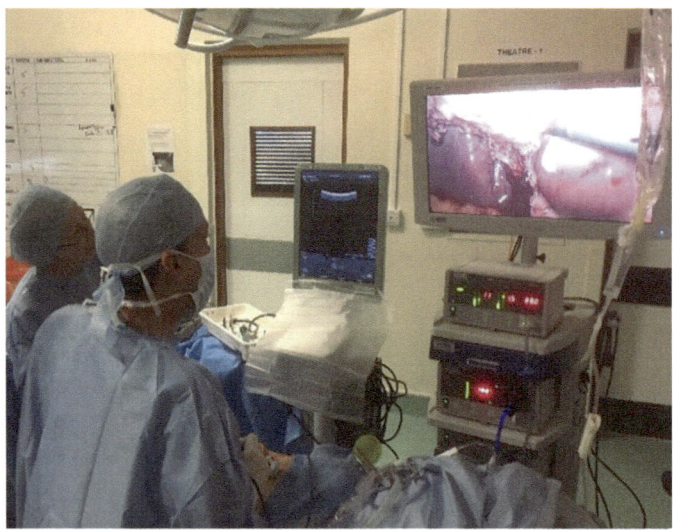

FIGURE 3.3 Laparoscopic ultrasound used during laparoscopy

Principles of Imaging Acquisition

If using sheaths for probes it is important to remember that ultrasonic gel is placed within the sheath around the transducer head in order to breakdown density interface picture quality problems.

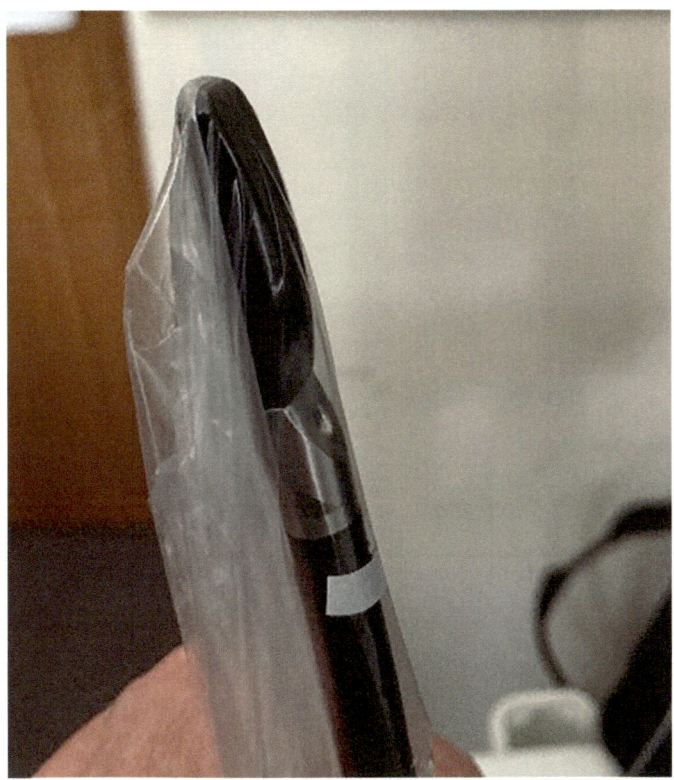

FIGURE 3.4 Laparoscopic ultrasound probe cover

The probe when inserted through the epigastric/left upper quadrant port will naturally rest on the porta hepatis in the short axis view to give cross-sectional view of the porta hepatis structures (Fig. 3.6). The ultrasound machine will rotate the image automatically so giving the user the impression that they are scanning the porta hepatis anteriorly to posterior (Fig. 3.6). This allows easier conceptualisation of imaging for the user.

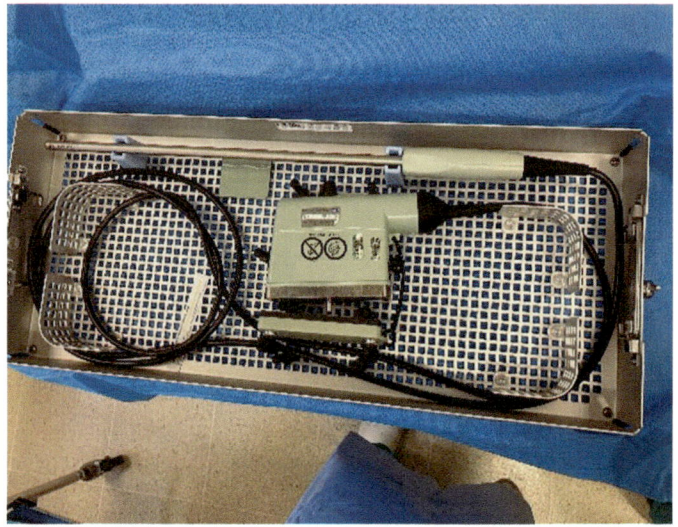

FIGURE 3.5 Laparoscopic ultrasound probe disinfected

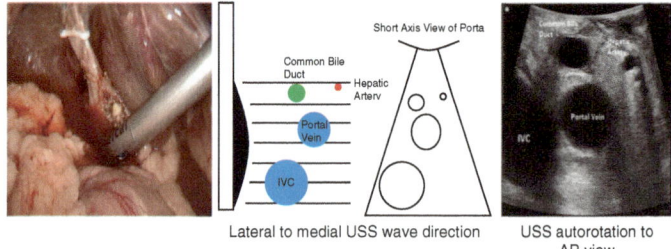

Lateral to medial USS wave direction   USS autorotation to AP view

FIGURE 3.6 Laparoscopic ultrasound probe resting on porta hepatis and images obtained. Lateral to medial USS wave direction; USS autorotation to AP view

Principles and Technique of Picture Acquisition

Acquiring information from LUS about the biliary tree that you trust to make decisions about patient care comes from a combination of training and experience in practice. Attending a training course and mentorship is advised.

We would recommend dissection of Calots triangle first, clipping and division of the cystic artery prior to performing the LUS. This allows greater access to the biliary system and manoeuvrability with the ultrasound probe around the porta hepatis structures. LUS is not the best modality for defining unclear biliary anatomy, if there is uncertainty, x-ray cholangiogram provides the best conformation.

Like any ultrasonic device media density interface degrades picture quality due to reflection which you must be mindful of, often there is sufficient moisture from tissue dissection alone for a high-quality image. However poor image quality can be improved with saline infusion intra-peritoneally pooling in sub-hepatic space to breakdown unwanted acoustic reflection (sometimes patient will need to be levelled from head up position). The probe is positioned perpendicular to the hepatoduodenal ligament on the porta hepatis, the linear array probe should immediately produce a cross-sectional image of the porta hepatis, 'the mickey mouse' view (Fig. 3.7). Grasping the gallbladder fundus with the left hand can provide additional manoverability and clarity of porta hepatis by lateral traction. **The vascular structures of the porta provide the navigation markers for clear identification of the CBD**. The colour doppler is activated on the ultrasound machine and doppler signal is confirmed using the doppler signal box in both the larger posterior structure -portal vein (mickey mouse face) and normally in screen right position- hepatic artery (mickey mouse left ear). No significant doppler signal is seen in common bile duct (mickey mouse right ear)

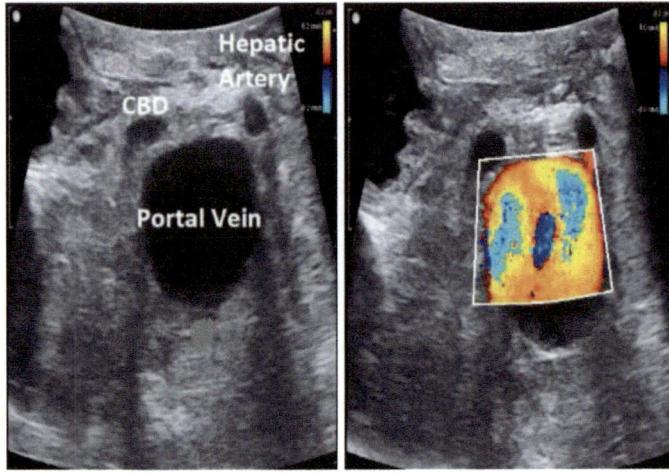

'Mickey Mouse View'   Doppler Signal on Portal Vein

FIGURE 3.7 The 'Mickey Mouse' view

(Fig. 3.8). Structures can vary in size and relative position within the porta hepatis so it is important to start each scan with this orientation procedure to be sure it is the biliary ductal system you are identifying. If you become lost during the scan process then returning to this default start point is advised.

Once the CBD is identified the aim is to travel inferiorly down the supra-duodenal bile duct keeping it central in position on the ultrasound image. The probe should rest gently on the hepatoduodenal ligament otherwise the CBD will be compressed and obscured, to little pressure and the ultrasound window on the porta will narrow.

The aim is to slowly and carefully examine the entire biliary drainage system from hepatic ducts to ampulla. It is important while manoeuvring the probe that you try and stay in the short axis plane producing crisp cross-sectional images to allow accurate interpretation. This is achieved with a combination of probe insertion and withdrawal and wrist rotation and has a learning curve. As the distal CBD passes through

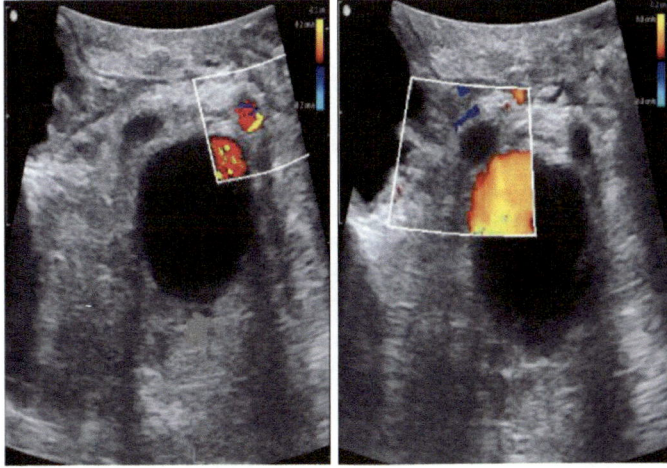

Doppler Signal Hepatic Artery   No Doppler Signal on CBD

FIGURE 3.8 Identification of hepatic artery and common bile duct. Doppler Signal on Portal Vein; Doppler Signal Hepatic Artery; No Doppler Signal on CBD

the pancreas it angulates laterally to join duodenum, in order to stay in short axis view of the CBD, reasonably significant supination of the wrist is required in combination with downwards travel of the probe to correctly angle the transducer (Fig. 3.9: a–c).

A complete scan involves several components and anatomical land marks can assist with this, they include right and left hepatic ducts and their confluence to form the common hepatic duct. Cystic duct and common hepatic duct confluence to form the CBD and pancreatic duct confluence with the CBD at the ampulla. The CBD should be followed down to its termination at the ampulla. The intra-pancreatic portion of the bile duct can sometimes be more difficult to interpret due to the echogenic reflectivity of the pancreas which can be made worse in patients with recent pancreatitis. A transduodenal view can sometimes help in this scenario (Fig. 3.10).

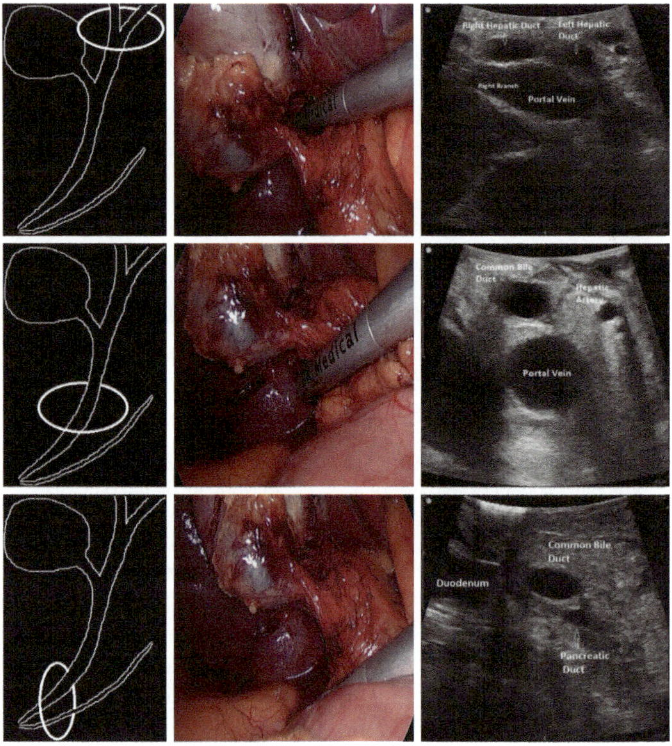

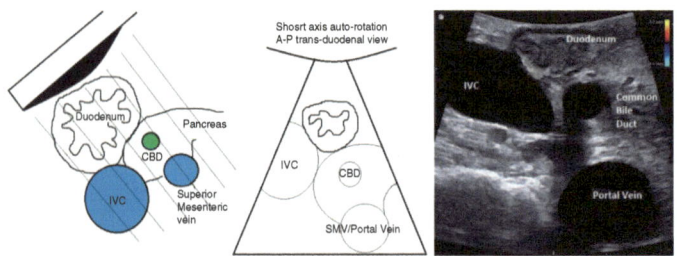

FIGURE 3.9 Downwards travel of the ultrasound probe; (**a**) Identification of left and right hepatic duct; (**b**) Identification of CBD 'Mickey Mouse View' (**c**) Identification of intra-pancreatic common bile duct and pancreatic duct

FIGURE 3.10 Trans-duodenal view of the common bile duct

Documentation and Pathology

It is good practice to document structures seen and take a standard set of measurements to record in the operation note, this involves using the measurement calliper function of the ultrasound machine to document CBD dimeter distally and proximally. It advisable to discuss with your x-ray department about linking the captured images from the ultrasound machine to the hospital radiology archive system.

Stones within the duct seen are usually very obvious with the casting of an acoustic shadow (Fig. 3.11). Echogenic sludge is sometimes seen within the duct system defined by its more diffuse appearance and lack of acoustic shadow and is usually of little clinical consequence and a CBD flush is recommended.

If using LUS for LCBDE then useful information can be obtained for surgical planning such as size of stone, CBD diameter and cystic duct diameter if attempting trans-cystic exploration (Fig. 3.12).

Business Case

Although the initial cost of equipment can seem high, cost analysis shows that equipment costs are covered after the first 60–70 cases of use based on cost of pre-operative MRCP

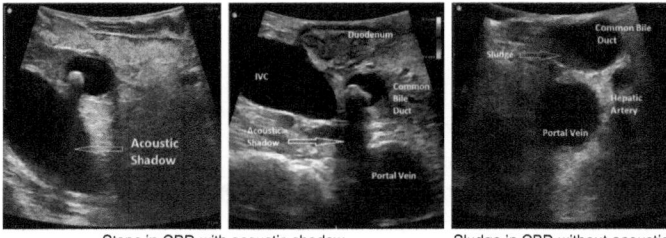

Stone in CBD with acoustic shadow   Sludge in CBD without acoustic shadow

FIGURE 3.11 Stones with and without acoustic shadow. Stone in CBD with acoustic shadow; Sludge in CBD without acoustic shadow

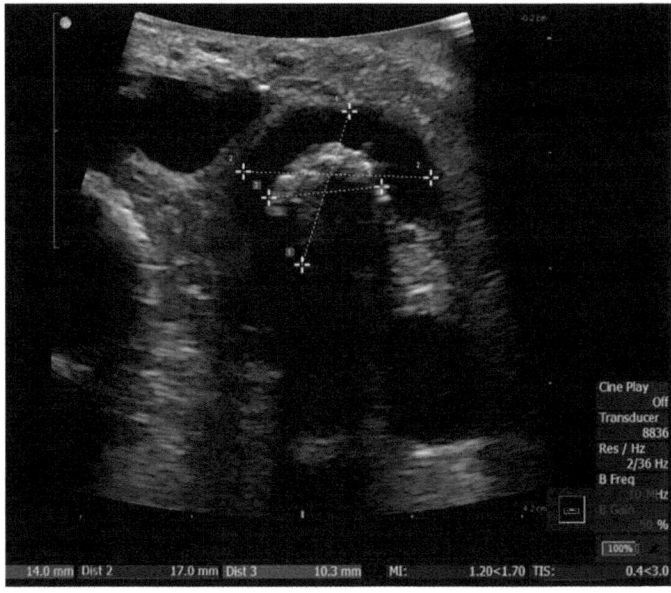

FIGURE 3.12 Assessing size stone

avoidance in both the inpatient or outpatient setting [9]. As patients presenting with symptomatic gallstones and synchronous deranged LFTs can procedure straight to surgery with the majority accurately reassured the bile duct is clear then emergency bed days can be saved through more efficient patient journey.

References

1. Costi R, Gnocchi A, Di Mario F, Sarli L. Diagnosis and management of choledocholithiasis in the golden age of imaging, endoscopy and laparoscopy. World J Gastroenterol. 2014;20(37):13382–401.
2. Aziz O, Ashrafian H, Jones C, Harling L, Kumar S, Garas G, et al. Laparoscopic ultrasonography versus intra-operative cholangiogram for the detection of common bile duct stones during laparoscopic cholecystectomy: a meta-analysis of diagnostic accuracy. Int J Surg. 2014;12(7):712–9.

3. Halpin VJ, Dunnegan D, Soper NJ. Laparoscopic intracorporeal ultrasound versus fluoroscopic intraoperative cholangiography: after the learning curve. Surg Endosc. 2002;16(2):336–41.
4. Perry KA, Myers JA, Deziel DJ. Laparoscopic ultrasound as the primary method for bile duct imaging during cholecystectomy. Surg Endosc. 2008;22(1):208–13.
5. Machi J, Oishi AJ, Tajiri T, Murayama KM, Furumoto NL, Oishi RH. Routine laparoscopic ultrasound can significantly reduce the need for selective intraoperative cholangiography during chole-cystectomy. Surg Endosc. 2007;21(2):270–4.
6. Jamal KN, Smith H, Ratnasingham K, Siddiqui MR, McLachlan G, Belgaumkar AP. Meta-analysis of the diagnostic accuracy of laparoscopic ultrasonography and intraoperative cholangiogra-phy in detection of common bile duct stones. Ann R Coll Surg Engl. 2016;98(4):244–9.
7. CholeS Study Group WsMRC. Population-based cohort study of outcomes following cholecystectomy for benign gallbladder dis-eases. Br J Surg. 2016;103(12):1704–15.
8. Sinha S, Hofman D, Stoker DL, Friend PJ, Poloniecki JD, Thompson MM, et al. Epidemiological study of provision of cho-lecystectomy in England from 2000 to 2009: retrospective analy-sis of hospital episode statistics. Surg Endosc. 2013;27(1):162–75.
9. Donoghue S, Jones RM, Bush A, Srinivas G, Bowling K, Andrews S. Cost effectiveness of intraoperative laparoscopic ultrasound for suspected choledocholithiasis; outcomes from a specialist benign upper gastrointestinal unit. Ann R Coll Surg Engl. 2020; https://doi.org/10.1308/rcsann.2020.0109.

Chapter 4
Equipment and Operative Setting for Laparoscopic Bile Duct Exploration (LBDE)

Alberto Martinez-Isla, María Asunción Acosta-Mérida, and Lalin Navaratne

Equipment

For laparoscopic bile duct exploration (LBDE) at the time of cholecystectomy, the standard laparoscopic cholecystectomy set can be complemented with disposable items listed in Table 4.1 and a 3 mm choledochoscope. Table 4.2 summarises the characteristics, advantages and disadvantages of the various 3 mm choledochoscopes currently available on the market. For complex choledocholithiasis, Lithotripsy Assisted Bile duct Exploration by Laparoendoscopy (LABEL) is

A. Martinez-Isla (✉) · L. Navaratne
Northwick Park and St Mark's Hospitals, London North West University Healthcare NHS Trust, London, UK
e-mail: a.isla@imperial.ac.uk; lalin.navaratne@doctors.org.uk

M. A. Acosta-Mérida
General Surgery Department, Hospital Universitario de Gran Canaria Doctor Negrín,
Las Palmas de Gran Canaria, Las Palmas, Spain

A. Martinez-Isla, L. Navaratne (eds.), *Laparoscopic Common Bile Duct Exploration*, In Clinical Practice,
https://doi.org/10.1007/978-3-030-93203-9_4

often required. The equipment required for LABEL will be discussed here, however, patient selection and technical aspects of LABEL will be described elsewhere (see Chap. 5).

Intra-Operative Cholangiogram (IOC)

In reality, transcystic LBDE begins with the cannulation of the cystic duct for intra-operative cholangiography (IOC). For cholangiography, we recommend using an open-end flexi-tip 5F (70 cm) catheter (Table 4.1, Serial 7) which can be introduced through a Horner needle (Table 4.1, Serial 1). Alternatively, if a Horner needle is not available, a disposable ENT suction device can be used to similar effect. An initial

TABLE 4.1 Disposable equipment

Serial	Item	Description	Picture
1	Steriseal Horner™ perioperative laparoscopic cholecystectomy cholangiogram set (Optech Diagnostic & Surgical)	Used to direct the catheter guidewire to the cystic duct opening	
2	Endoloop® (Ethicon) or Surgitie™ (Covidien)	For retraction of the proximal cystic duct	
3	Endo close™ trocar site closure device (Covidien)	To retract the Endoloop® or Surgitie™ through the anterior abdominal wall	

TABLE 4.1 (continued)

Serial	Item	Description	Picture
4	Adjustable biopsy Port sealing device (Olympus)	Used to make the working channel watertight. Can be connected to [8] if needed	
5	2.4F (120 cm) Dormia basket (cook medical) or 2.4F (120 cm) Segura hemisphere™ retrieval basket (Boston Scientific)	For CBD stone extraction	
6	Flexor® ureteral access sheath 9.5-12F (35 cm) (cook medical)	To introduce 3 mm choledochoscope	
7	Open-end flexi-tip® 5F (70 cm) catheter (cook medical)	To cannulate the cystic duct and perform intraoperative cholangiogram	
8	3-way valve	Allows dual use of the working channel for irrigation and basket instrumentation	
9	Ureteral dilator set 6-18F (cook medical)	To achieve cystic duct dilatation and introduce 5 mm scope	
10	PTFE guidewire (0.035 inch diameter, 145 cm length, 3 cm flexible tip) (cook medical)	The catheter [7] and dilator [6] can be railroaded over the guidewire for access	

TABLE 4.2 Summary of the characteristics and advantages of the different 3 mm choledochoscopes available

	Cost per case	Diameter	Quality	Sterilization	Steering	Maintenance	Availability	Working channel	Deflection	Additional stack required
SpyGlass™ discover (Boston Scientific)	£££	3.5 mm	+++	N/A	4-way	N/A	+++	3.6F	++++	No
Disposable PUSEN	££	3 mm	++	N/A	2-way	N/A	+++	3.6F	+++	No
Disposable AMBU®	£	3 mm	+	N/A	2-way	N/A	+++	3.6F	+	No
Reusable Fibreoptic	££	3 mm	++	Complex	2-way	Complex	+	3.6F	++	Yes
Reusable Digital	£££	3 mm	+++	Complex	2-way	Complex	+	3.6F	++	Yes

attempt should be made to introduce the catheter directly into the cystic duct. In some patients, the tortuosity of the cystic duct and/or the spiral valves of Heister prevent easy passage of the cholangiocatheter. In such cases, a guidewire (Table 4.1, Serial 10) can be used to railroad the catheter safely into the common bile duct (CBD) [1]. Once the cholangiogram is completed, and if LBDE is indicated, the guidewire is reintroduced through the 5F Cholangiocatheter. The cystic duct can be gently dilated by railroading a 9.5-12F Flexor® Ureteral Access Sheath (Cook Medical, Bloomington, IN, USA) (Table 4.1, Serial 6) over the guidewire. This manoeuvre has dual purpose, as the inner sheath dilates the cystic duct as mentioned, and the outer sheath can introduce the 3 mm choledochoscope. The access sheath is hydrophilic and therefore should be wet prior to its introduction.

Retraction of the Liver

Complex laparoscopic upper gastrointestinal procedures may necessitate the use of the Nathanson retractor for retraction of the left lobe of the liver (Fig. 4.1). We advocate using the French technique (or double-access position) for positioning of the patient during cholecystectomy and LBDE (Fig. 4.2) [2]. In this position, the hook of the Nathanson retractor is introduced through the 5 mm epigastric port incision (after removal of the port). We find that this retraction provides excellent exposure of the hilum when combined with our preferred positioning of the patient (Figs. 4.1, 4.2 and 4.3). If the surgeon is concerned about the risks associated with insertion of the Nathanson liver retractor (bleeding, haematoma formation or creating of false tracts), an alternative technique of safe insertion using a 12F Jacques Nelaton catheter (Teleflex Medical, High Wycomb, UK) as a 'guidewire' has been described [3]; in our experience this has never been necessary but we think that it is an useful trick to know.

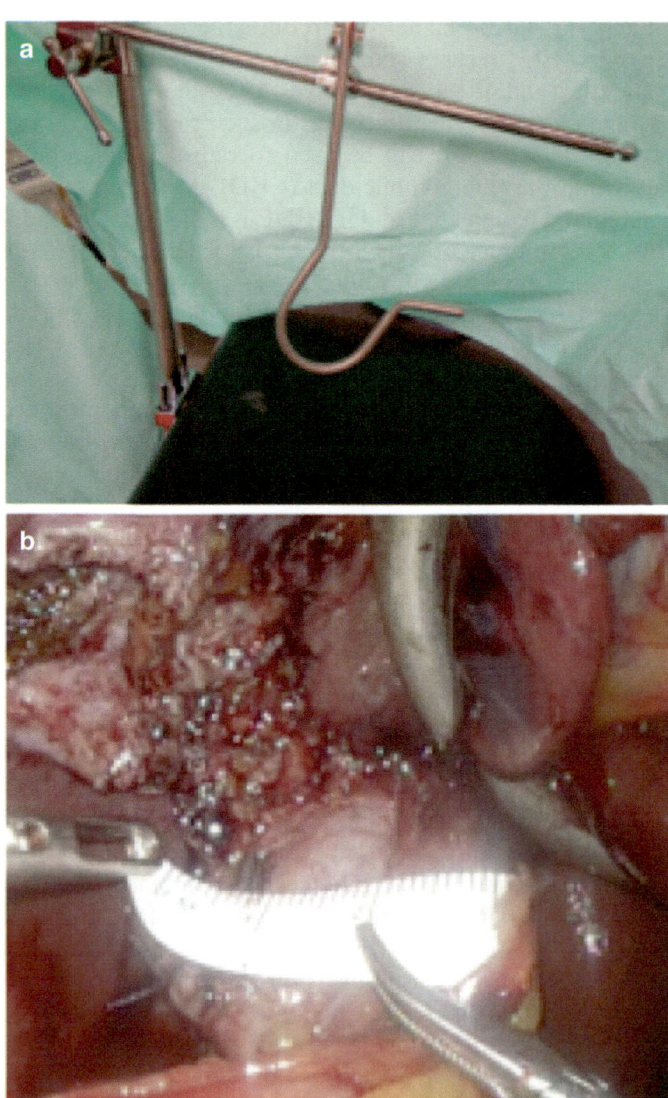

FIGURE 4.1 (**a**) Nathanson liver retractor. (**b**) intraoperative measurement of the CBD

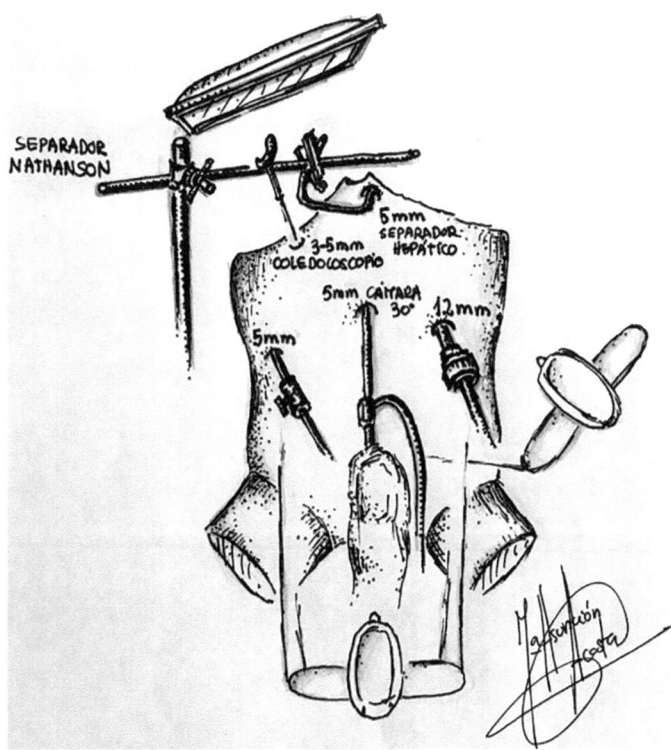

FIGURE 4.2 Surgical setting

Choledochoscopes

Flexible choledochoscopes are a crucial part of the equipment required for LBDE. Choledochoscopes are available in two sizes: 3 mm and 5 mm, and are similar to cystoscopes and ureteroscopes, but require a different method of sterilisation. The video image can be digital or fibreoptic, the former providing better picture quality and not subject to deterioration due to rupturing of the fibres. Furthermore, an additional camera will not be necessary for digital choledochoscopes. Like other endoscopes, choledochoscopes have a working channel for guidewires, baskets, lithotripsy probes etc. The

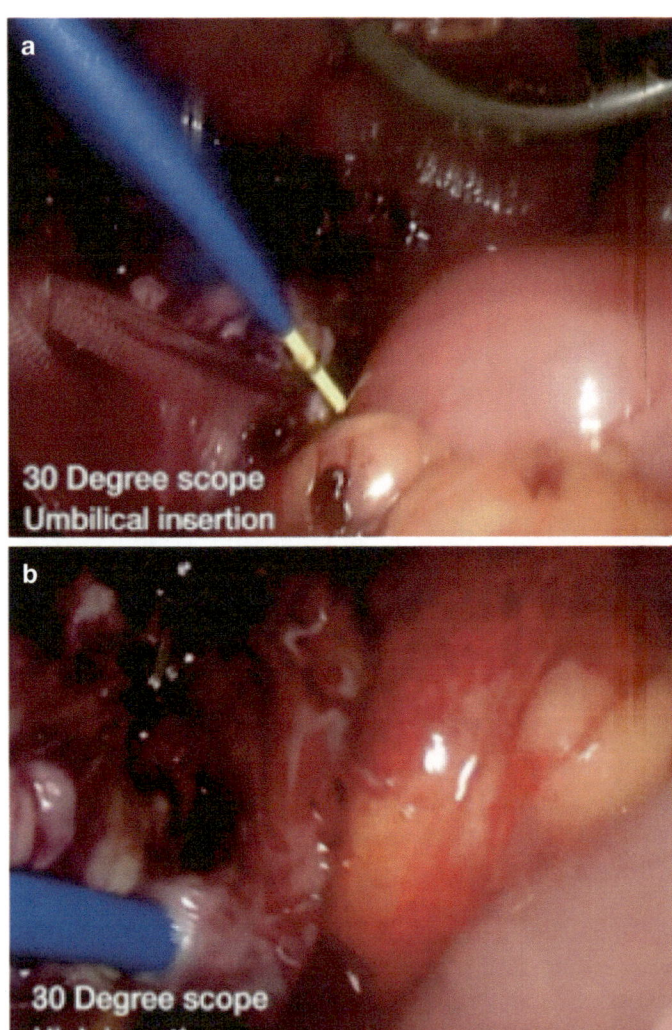

FIGURE 4.3 Views of the CBD with a 30° laparoscope from different port sites. (**a**) At the umbilicus. (**b**) Epigastric

working channel in a 5 mm choledochoscope is up to 6F and 2.5-3.6F in a 3 mm choledochoscope. Choledochoscopes can be reusable or single-use (disposable). Reusable 3 mm scopes, whether digital or fibreoptic, are very delicate and break easily. In the best-case scenario, you can expect a maximum of 20–30 uses before a technical fault which may require costly and lengthy repairs. Reusable scopes also need to be sterilised, which is costly and often needs to be performed on an alternative site. For a relatively busy service, performing one to two LBDEs per week, we recommend stocking a minimum of three choledochoscopes if the institutional preference is for using reusable choledochoscopes. Historically, most disposable scopes were in fact ureteroscopes, not specifically designed for use in the bile duct. Figure 4.4a demonstrates the use of the PUSEN ureteroscope (Zhuhai PUSEN Medical Technology Co., Ltd., China) during LBDE. Recently Boston Scientific has launched the SpyGlass™ Discover (Fig. 4.4b), which is a 3.5 mm specifically designed disposable (single-use) choledochoscope. It has a 3.6F working channel and the two-wheel control offers four-way steering, similar to a gastroscope or colonoscope, allowing superior tip control. This is particularly important during lithotripsy, when precision targeting of the CBD stone is essential for safety and treatment success. The disposable scope also comes equipped with an accessory suction irrigation channel which can be also used as an extra irrigation channel during lithotripsy. The working channel is independent this avoids retrograde fluid spilling during the procedure. The SpyGlass™ Discover can be introduced through a 12F ureteral sheath (refer to table) with the dilator to aid cannulation of the cystic duct once railroaded over the guidewire. We had the opportunity of being the first European team to use the new SpyGlass™ Discover in a live patient. The four-way steering allows precise targeting and relies less on excessive torque and therefore more natural movements. Other disposable scopes (particularly ureteroscopes) equipped with two-way steering require more torque, which can result in detachment of the tip from shaft of the scope thereby breaking it; moreover, the irrigation shares the

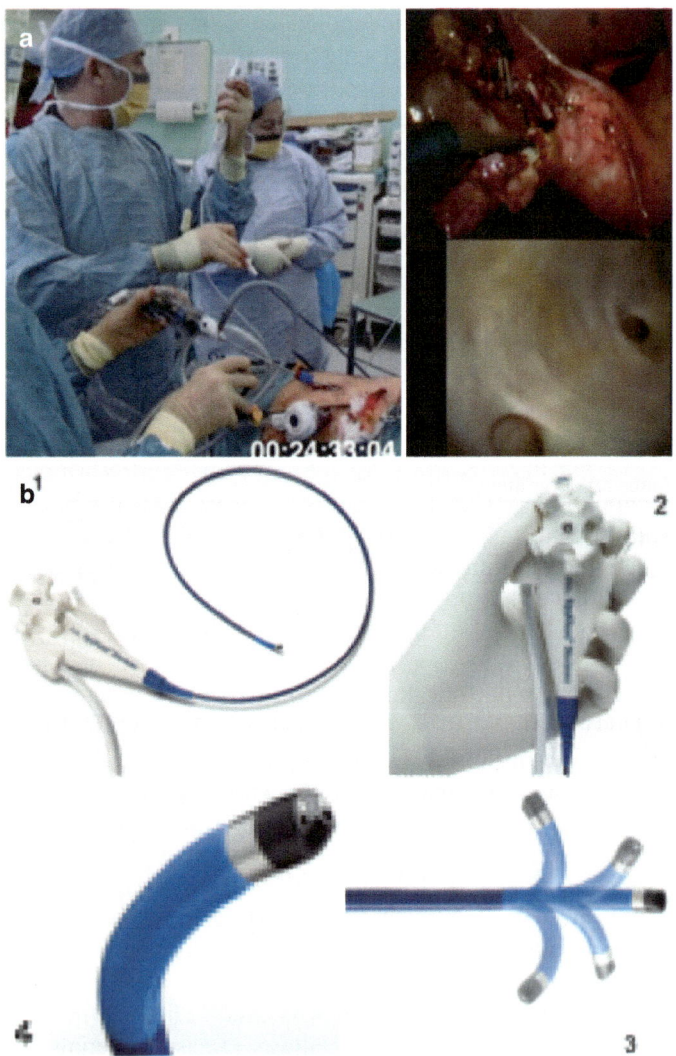

FIGURE 4.4 3 mm disposable choledochoscopes. (a) PUSEN uretero-scope. (b) SpyGlass™ Discover Boston Scientific

working channel making necessary the use of a biopsy port to avoid unpleasant fluid spillage on the face during the procedure. Table 4.2 summarises the characteristics, advantages and disadvantages of the various 3 mm choledochoscopes currently available on the market.

Scope Fatigue

With prolonged usage times, the performance of both disposable and reusable choledochoscopes will drop. We describe this phenomenon as *scope fatigue*. Reusable digital choledochoscopes are least likely to become troubled with this, whereas reusable fibreoptic choledochoscopes can show fatigue with use manifested by the appearance of black dots on the video display corresponding to broken optic fibres. In our experience, disposable choledochoscopes are also likely to experience fatigue with prolonged use. The most commonly observed problems are loosening of the junction between the deflecting tip and the shaft of the scope (thereby losing the ability to transmit torque to the tip), general degradation of the deflecting mechanism over time and peeling of the outer plastic cover of the scope shaft. We have also noticed that introducing the laser fibre (stiff) with the scope in deflection has led to perforation of the working channel and exteriorization of the fibre through the lateral side of the scope. Injection of lubrication jelly into the working channel of the choledochoscope may help. When using laser lithotripsy with both disposable and reusable choledochoscopes, it is very important not to activate the laser inside of the working channel as this will damage the scope. Scope fatigue is more likely to affect disposable scopes, however, in the vast majority of cases, a single disposable choledochoscope will be sufficient to do the job.

Scope Failure

Scope failure is the inability to continue a bile duct exploration due to a malfunctioning scope. Possible causes of scope

failure include complete disruption of the video display/
image, the inability to manoeuvre the scope due to malfunctioning tip deflection, light source failure and damage to the
optical fibres by heavy handed grasping of the shaft of a reusable 3 mm choledochoscope. During long procedures it may
be necessary to change the scope. We have had to use three
disposable choledochoscopes in a single operation for a
patient with complex type II Mirizzi syndrome which required
more than 7 h of lithotripsy. Scope fatigue and failure appears
to affect disposable scopes more frequently, however, the cost
effectiveness of using multiple disposable scopes versus send-
ing an expensive reusable choledochoscope for repair (which
can be very costly and place the scope out of action for several weeks) needs to be considered when setting up a new
service.

Laser Lithotripsy

Light activation by the stimulated emission of radiation
(LASER) technology has been utilised for the treatment of
urinary stones since the mid-1980s. Two laser devices that are
in use today for the endoscopic treatment of CBD stones are
the frequency-doubled double-pulse neodymium:YAG
(FREDDY) and holmium:YAG (holmium) lasers. The mechanism of action of these lasers differ, thereby producing different safety and efficacy profiles. FREDDY laser lithotripsy
causes fragmentation of the stone by the generation of a
plasma bubble with mechanical shockwave effects, whereas
holmium laser lithotripsy uses a photothermal mechanism of
action by creating a vapour bubble that transmits laser energy
[4–6]. There have been no studies to date comparing these
two modalities during LCBDE. However, in one study comparing FREDDY and holmium lasers during ureteroscopic
lithotripsy, the two modalities demonstrated similar stone-
free and complication rates, though there was a trend toward
a higher complication rate and lower stone-free rate with the
FREDDY laser [4]. The two lasers have similar start-up costs

TABLE 4.3 Description of the costs associated with purchase of the devices and fibres for laser lithotripsy

Laser modality	Device Cost	Fibre cost
Holmium	£50,000	£300–£500 (200 μm)
FREDDY	£45,000	£280–£480 (280 μm)

All fibres are disposable

(i.e., device purchase costs) and laser fibre costs (Table 4.3). At the authors institution, holmium laser lithotripsy is preferred, and due to its widespread use in urological procedures, the laser system (device) should already be available in most hospitals [5, 7]. The laser fibres are disposable and cost approximately £400 (€450) and are available in different diameters. We recommend the 200 μm because it is the smallest and therefore will have less impact on deflecting the tip of the scope. There is no official accreditation to be able to use laser lithotripsy, but several laser safety courses are available to become familiar with the equipment and safety protocols. Figure 4.5 shows a laser safety checklist which is in use at our institution. Use of the laser lithotripsy device (Fig. 4.6a) must be conducted in a laser-amenable operating theatre which has been fitted with the appropriate electrical sockets and blinds (Fig. 4.6b, c). Therefore, when faced with the possibility of managing complex CBD stones (see Chap. 5, section "Which Patients Might Require LABEL?": Which patients might require LABEL?), an appropriate operating theatre should be booked that can cater for use of laser lithotripsy. Additionally, it is important to be aware that different lasers have different wavelengths and each will require the specific protection goggles for that particular wavelength (Fig. 4.6d).

Electrohydraulic Lithotripsy (EHL)

The AUTOLITH® TOUCH (Northgate technologies Inc., Elgin, IL, USA) Bipolar Electrohydraulic Lithotripter (EHL) is a software controlled, electronic device capable of fragmenting biliary calculi of any size and composition (Fig. 4.7).

Laser Safety Checklist

Laser machine pre-checked and calibrated including delivery device?

Yes ☐   No: ....

All doors closed and blinds down?

Yes ☐   No: ....

Laser warning light outside each door of theatre is switched ON?

Yes ☐   No: ....

Protective eyewear warn by all staff in theatre, except for surgeon performing the procedure with filtered microscope laser?
(Only ENT)

Yes ☐   No: ....

Laser mask warn by all staff?

Yes ☐   No: ....

Jug of saline available on scrub trolley?

Yes ☐   No: ....

Patient's eyes protected with laser eye shields?
(Only ENT)

Yes ☐   No: ....

Wet gauze used to protect patient's face and neck?
(Only ENT)

Yes ☐   No: ....

Location of fire extinguisher known?

Yes ☐   No: ....

Laser register book to be completed at the end of the procedure.

Yes ☐   No: ....

FIGURE 4.5 Laser safety checklist

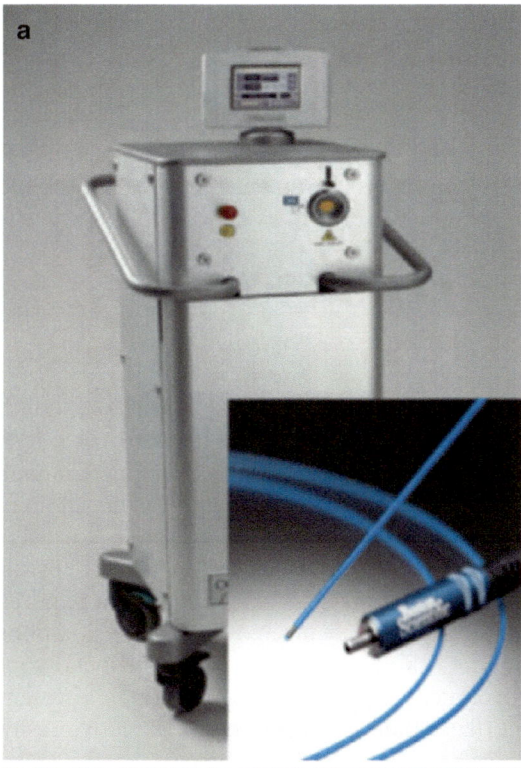

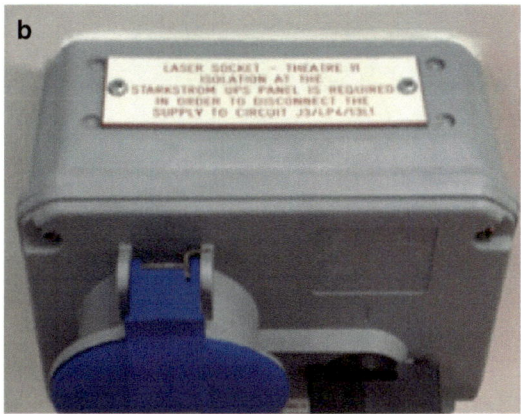

FIGURE 4.6 Equipment required for LABEL. (**a**) laser generator and probe. (**b**) special electrical socket. (**c**) theatre blinds. (**d**) goggles

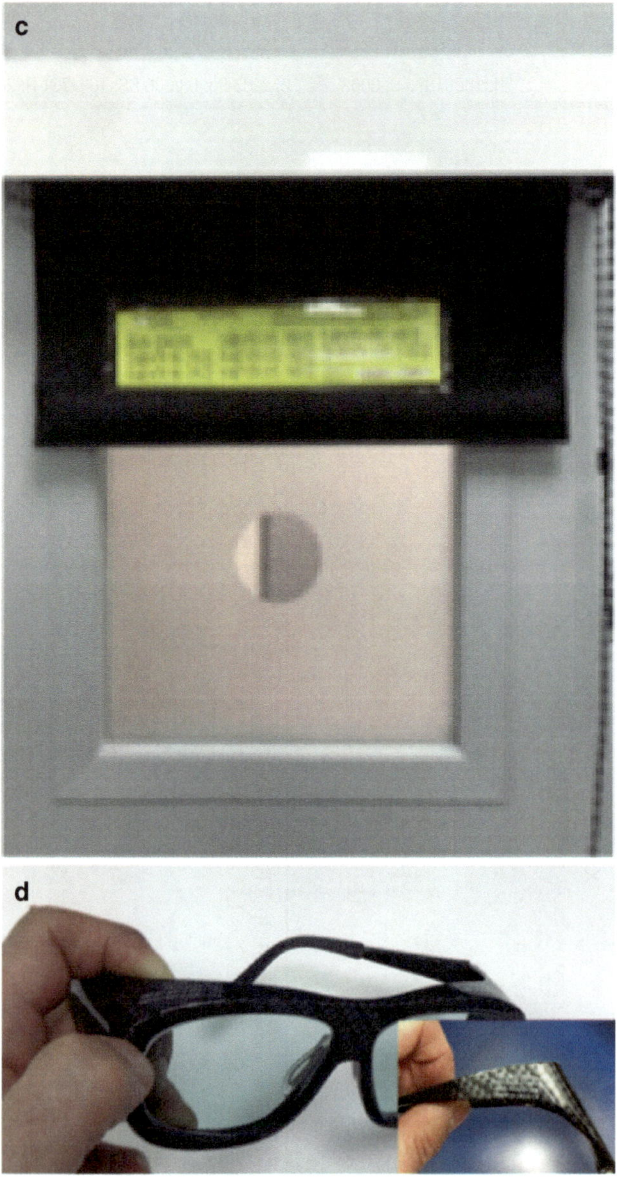

c

d

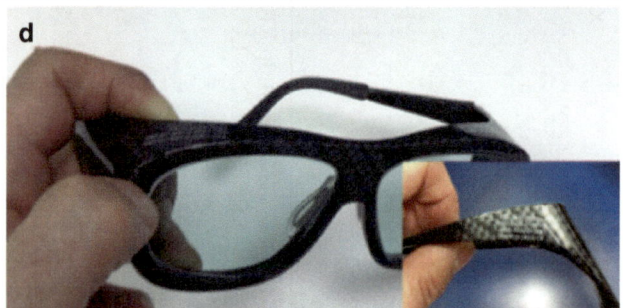

FIGURE 4.6 (continued)

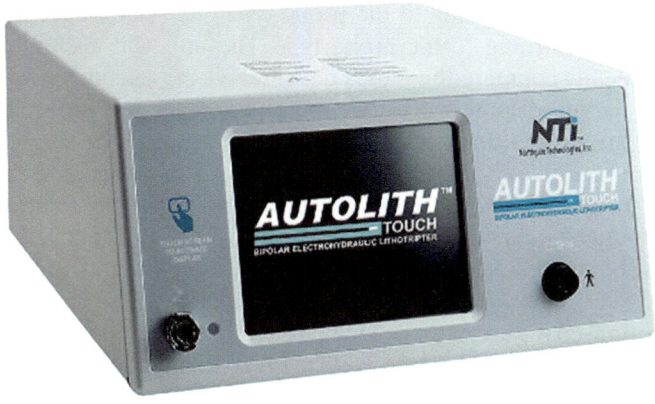

FIGURE 4.7 The AUTOLITH® TOUCH (Northgate technologies Inc., Elgin, IL, USA) Bipolar Electrohydraulic Lithotripter (EHL) unit

The electronic circuitry generates a single high-voltage pulse or a series of pulses across the tip of a flexible bipolar lithotripter probe. When discharged in 0.9% normal saline solution, these pulses produce sharp, high-amplitude hydraulic shock waves that fragment calculi located within the bile duct. The components of this device are:

- AUTOLITH® TOUCH unit
- Operation/Maintenance Manual
- Extender cable
- Foot Switch
- Detachable Power Cord

The AUTOLITH® TOUCH unit is a software controlled, lithotripter device and will regulate the discharge voltage and repetition rate of a shot delivered to a connected extender cable and probe. The unit will display the relative power delivered to the probe, the number of pulses to be delivered to the probe as requested by the surgeon and the number of pulses delivered. The unit will automatically sense the existence of a plugged-in probe, preset start-up values for power and pulses according to the probe type and scale the power range according to the probe type. The unit will also automatically compare the pulses delivered at the selected power levels and display when to inspect or replace the probe. To ensure proper operation of the EHL unit during the surgical procedure, 0.9% normal saline must be used to irrigate the endoscopic viewing field, and no other irrigating solution should be used. The AUTOLITH® TOUCH 1.9F 375 cm EHL Probe is a single-use device and is to be used with the AUTOLITH® TOUCH EHL unit. The EHL probe has been optimised for use with the SpyGlass™ DS Direct Visualisation System (Boston Scientific, Natick, MA, USA) to help manage large biliary stones. EHL is contraindicated in patients who have an externally connected intra-cardiac catheter or pacemaker.

Operative Setting

Patient Position

Prior to induction of general anaesthesia, all patients should be consented according to local and/or national guidelines (e.g. GMC guidelines in the UK) [8]. For laparoscopic cholecystectomy ± LBDE, we prefer the French position with the surgeon standing between the legs [2]. As previously mentioned, in complex cases or in patients with large fatty livers we may use a Nathanson retractor to retract the liver (Figs. 4.1 and 4.2) [9–12]. During choledochoscopy, the choledochoscope is handled by the surgeon with their left hand and the Dormia basket with their right hand. Opening and closing of the basket is performed by either the first assistant (standing to the patient's left side) or the second assistant/scrub nurse (standing to the patient's right side). The monitors for the choledochoscope and laparoscope are displayed to the right of the head-end of the operating table as shown in Fig. 4.2.

Port Placement

At the authors institution, positioning of the ports has evolved since 1998 when the first LBDE was performed until now (Fig. 4.2) [10, 11]. The most significant change was realised after moving the position of the 5 mm 30° laparoscope. Previously, this was placed at the umbilicus, but a superior view of the CBD is obtained if it is placed more cranially, some 15 cm below the xiphoid (Fig. 4.3). An optimal view of the CBD is especially important in more challenging cases (e.g. fibrotic and/or inflamed hilum) or obese patients with a long xipho-umbilical distance [12]. The improved view of the CBD and hilum is more in keeping with the view experienced during the open era of CBD exploration. The surgeon's right hand provides laparoscopic instrumentation through a 10–12 mm port in the patient's left upper quadrant (approximately in the midclavicular line and horizontally level with the laparoscope port). The surgeon's left hand operates another laparoscopic instrument through a 5 mm port in the patient's right flank. A high 5 mm epigastric port (near the xiphoid) is used for retracting the gallbladder fundus by the assistant's right hand or the Nathanson liver retractor as previously discussed. Finally, if choledochoscopy is indicated, an extra 5 mm port can be inserted in the right upper quadrant for a 5 mm scope or a 12F sheath for a 3–3.5 mm choledochoscope.

Cholecystectomy

Exposure of Calot's triangle and cystic artery ligation should be performed in the standard way. Following dissection of Calot's triangle, we find that there are two key steps that facilitate transcystic intubation. The first step is to mobilise the gallbladder from the liver bed without transecting the cystic duct. The second step is to completely dissect the cystic duct all the way to the cystobiliary junction. The application of an Endoloop® (Ethicon, New Brunswick, New Jersey,

USA) or Surgitie™ (Covidien, Mansfield, Massachusetts, USA) at the infundibulum, which is then exteriorised through the abdominal wall in the right upper quadrant using an Endo Close™ (Covidien, Mansfield, Massachusetts, USA), allows a 45° horizontal elevation (Fig. 4.8) and ideally a perpendicular cystic duct relative to the CBD [13]. Figure 4.9 demonstrates our 'gallbladder mobilisation first' approach

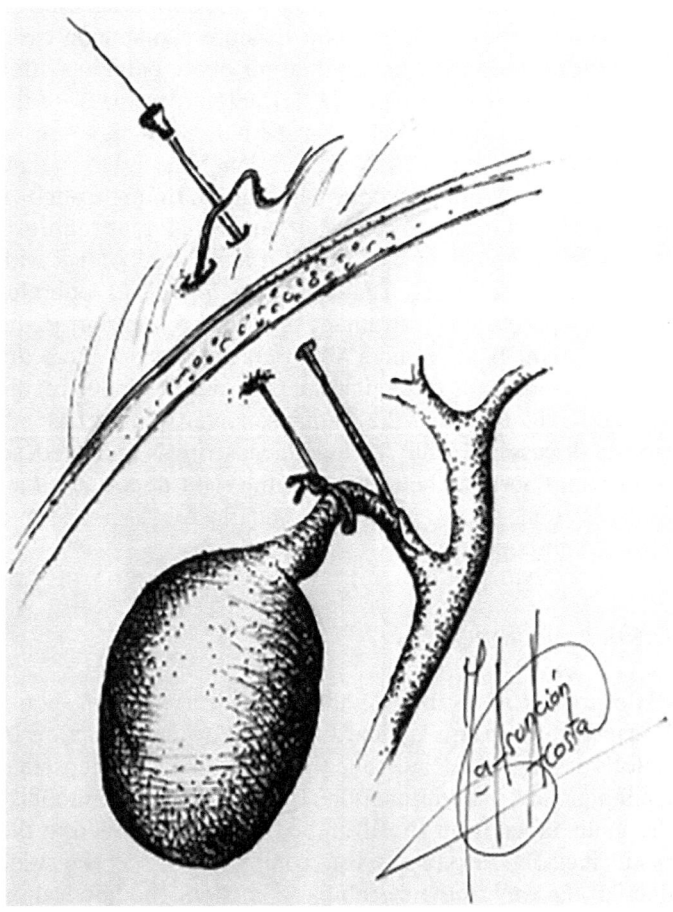

FIGURE 4.8 Retraction of the proximal cystic duct with an Endoloop

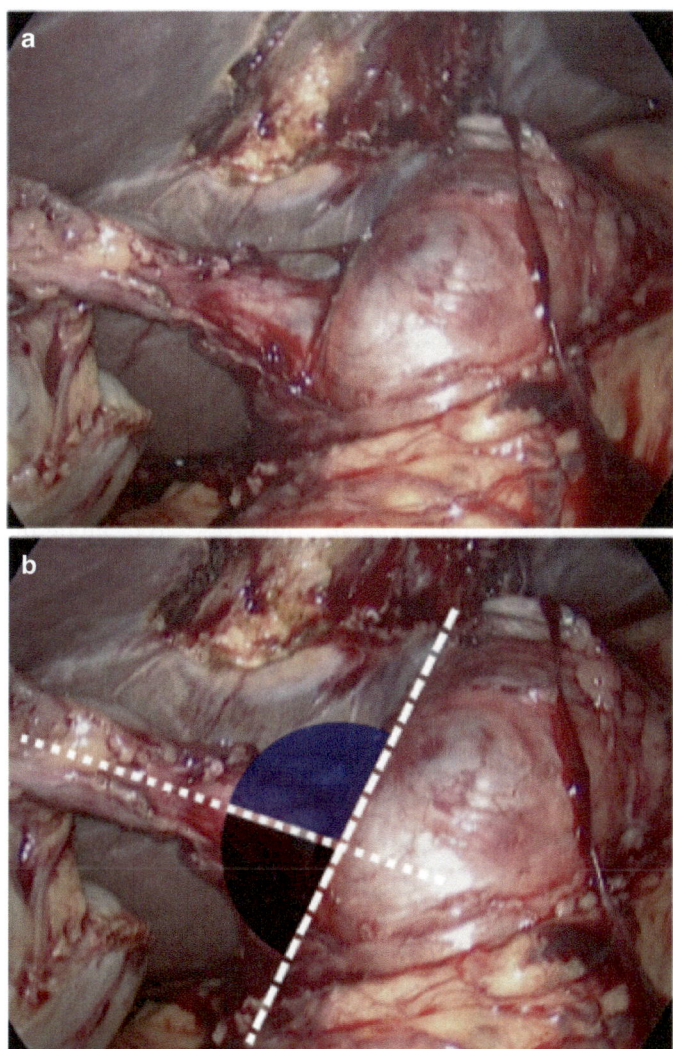

FIGURE 4.9 Correction of cystic duct-common bile duct angle. (**a**) Dissection of the gallbladder from the liver. (**b**) Creation of ~90° angle. (**c, d**) Endoloop retraction. (**e**) Determining optimal angle for traction (white arrow: extracorporeal palpation). (**f, g**) Exteriorising the Endoloop. (**h**) Guidewire cannulation of the cystic duct. (**i**) Choledochoscopy with 5 mm scope

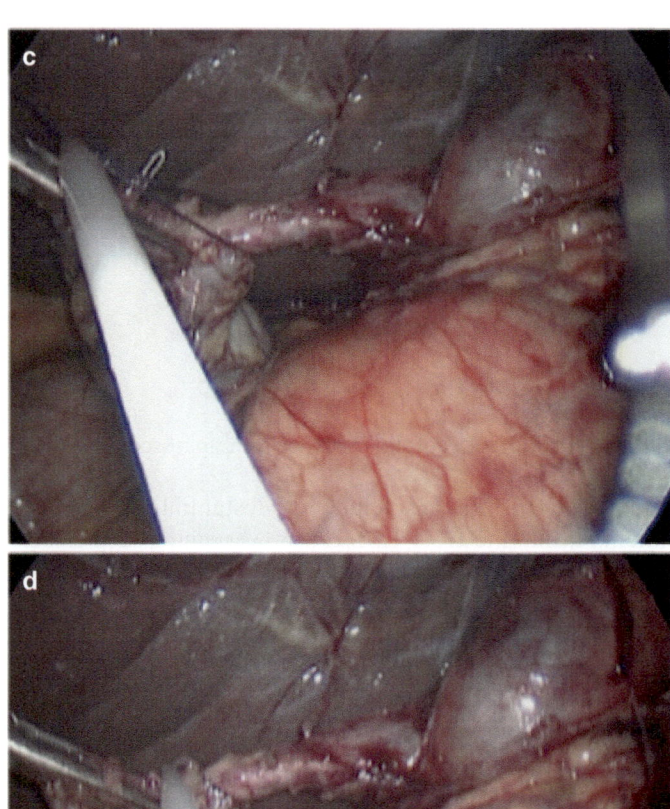

FIGURE 4.9 (continued)

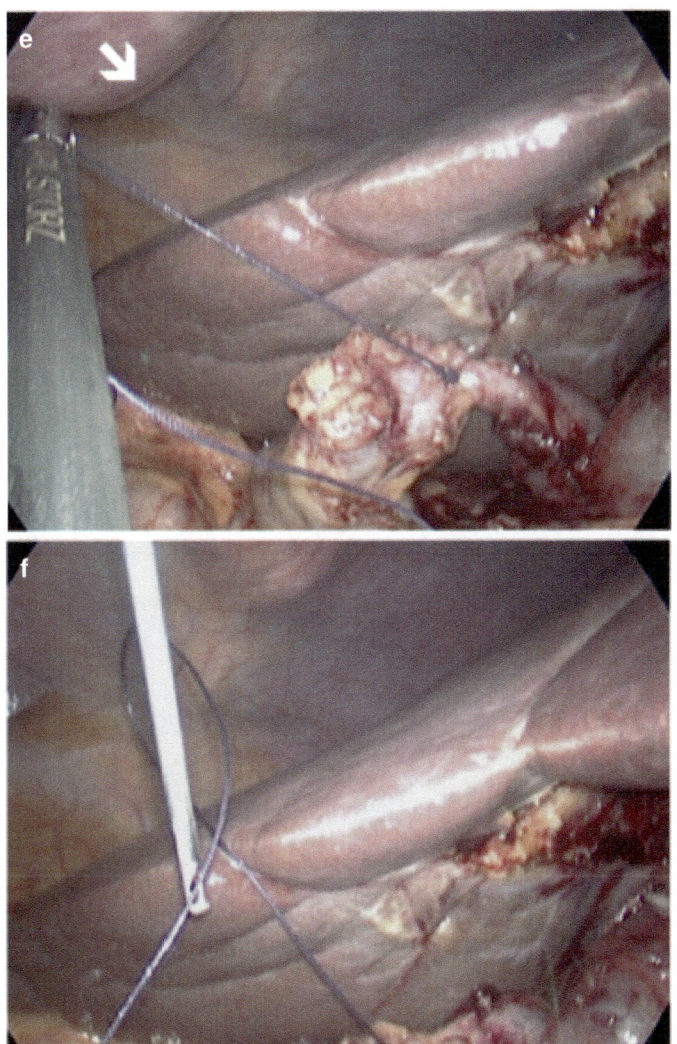

FIGURE 4.9 (continued)

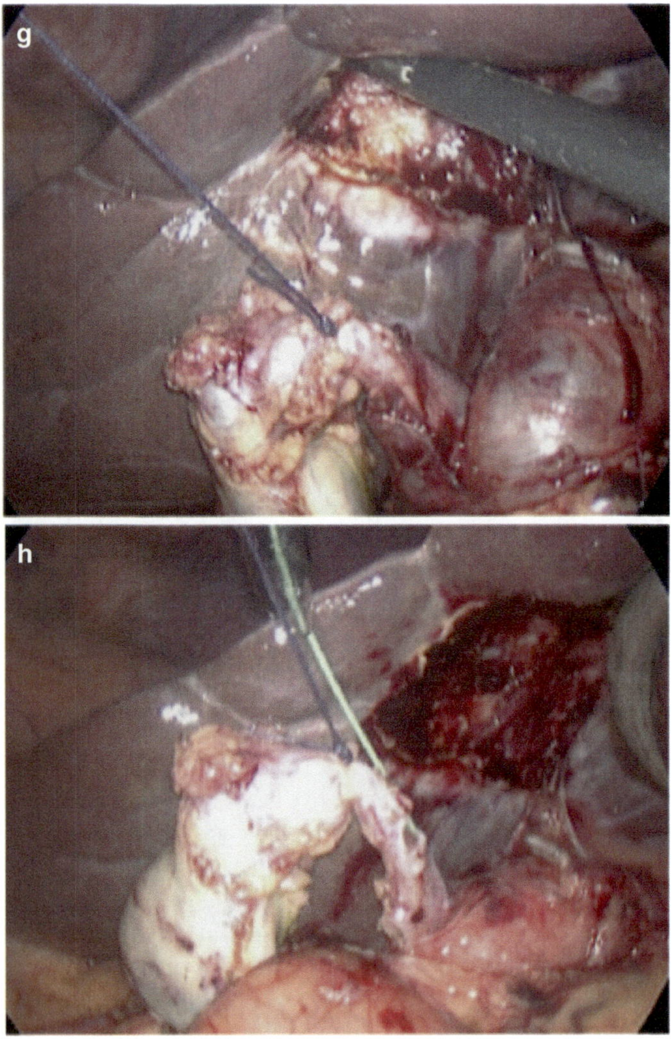

FIGURE 4.9 (continued)

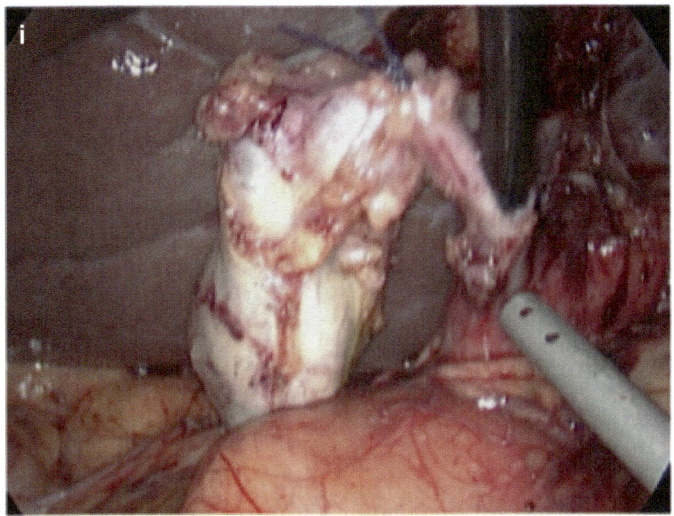

FIGURE 4.9 (continued)

resulting in correction of the cystic duct-common bile duct angle to a more favourable ~90°. A small incision is then made in the cystic duct to provide access for intra-operative cholangiogram and/or transcystic choledochoscopy.

Intra-Operative Cholangiogram (IOC)

Choledocholithiasis is a dynamic disease and as there is constant passage of stone material, we believe that an MRI performed days or weeks before surgical intervention does not guarantee that the bile duct is going to be clear on the day of cholecystectomy. For this reason, the CBD should be assessed intraoperatively with intra-operative cholangiogram (IOC) or laparoscopic intra-operative ultrasound (LIOUS). The need for contemporary imaging is illustrated in Fig. 4.10, which demonstrates pre-operative diagnosis of multiple CBD stones on MRCP (Fig. 4.10a) but normal choledochoscopy (with a widely open papilla) in the same patient at the time

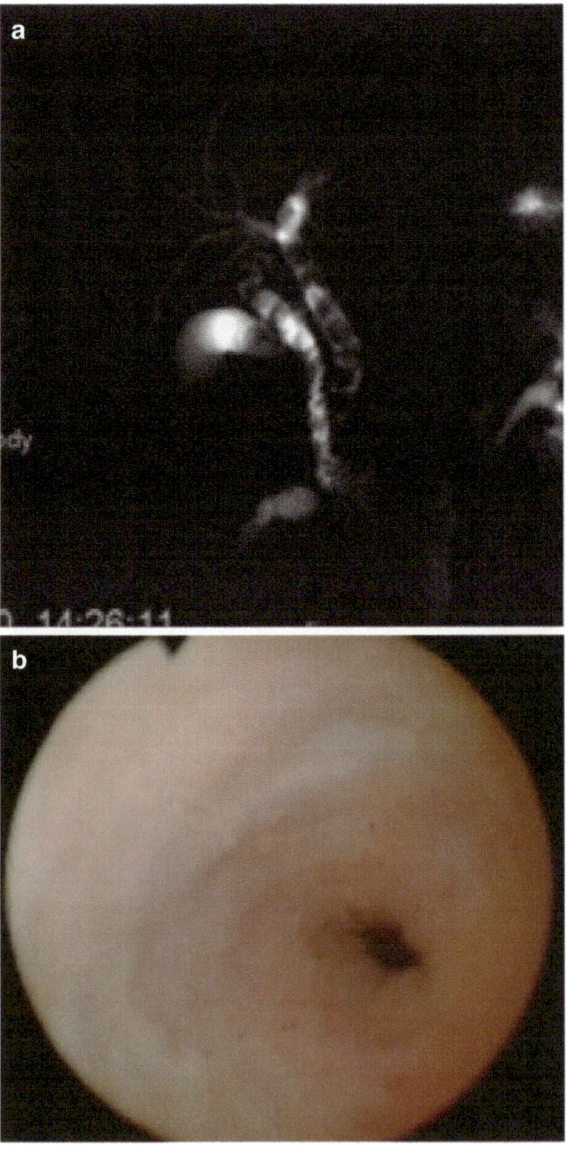

FIGURE 4.10 (a) MRCP demonstrating multiple CBD stones. (b) cholangioscopy demonstrating no CBD stones

of surgery (Fig. 4.10b). In patients with a high index of suspicion, or in patients who are pregnant or allergic to iodine, a sensible approach is to perform LIOUS or proceed directly to 3 mm transcystic choledochoscopy.

Once an incision has been made in the cystic duct, the cholangiogram needle can be introduced through the abdominal wall in the right upper quadrant. We recommend using the Horner needle (Table 4.1, Serial 1), however, if one is not available then a Belluci style 30° ENT disposable suction tube can be used instead (Fig. 4.11). If an ENT disposable suction tube is used, the 30° angulation in the tube needs to be straightened out, which can be done easily by hand. For easier cannulation, an attempt should be made to align the cholangiogram needle (or ENT suction tube) with the axis of the cystic duct (Fig. 4.12). An open-end Flexi-Tip® 5F (70 cm) catheter (Cook Medical) (Table 4.1, Serial 7) can then be introduced through the needle into the cystic duct. If the cannulation is challenging, a PTFE guidewire (0.035-inch diameter, 145 cm length, 3 cm flexible tip) (Cook Medical) (Table 4.1, Serial 10) can be used to cannulate the cystic duct, and thereafter, the 5F catheter can be railroaded over the guidewire. The catheter can be secured with a single clip, however, it may impede the flow of contrast during the cholangiogram and may also prevent its use as a working channel if the surgeons wants to perform the basket-in-catheter (BIC) technique for transcystic access to the bile duct [14]. Our preference is not to use it.

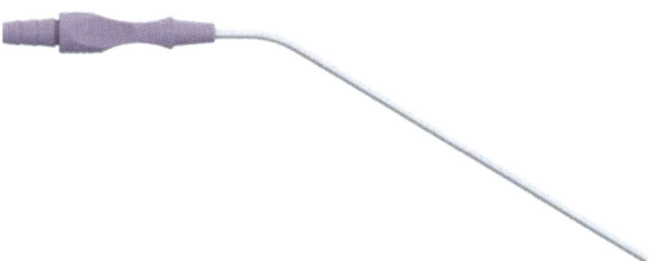

FIGURE 4.11 Belluci style 30° ENT disposable suction tube

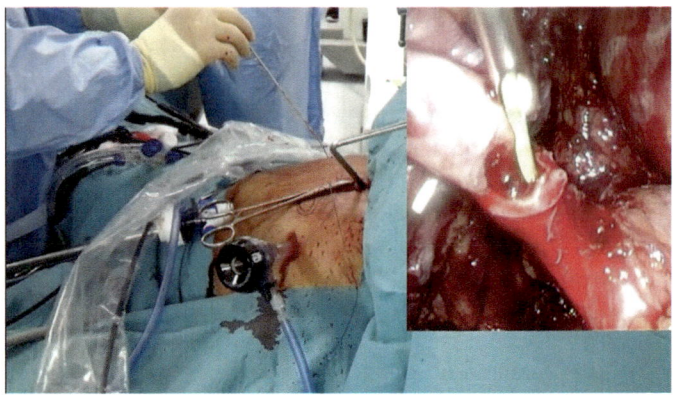

FIGURE 4.12 Cannulation of a guidewire into the cystic duct using a Horner's needle

For IOC we use Omnipaque™ (iohexol) 300 mg I/ml (GE Healthcare, Oslo, Norway) and a mobile C-arm. The correct sequence for obtaining a cholangiogram can be remembered by the pneumonic '**COAX**'. The first step ('C') ensures that the **C**lips appear in the **C**entre of the image. The second step ('O') involves **O**rientation of the image (Fig. 4.13). The spinous processes of the thoracic spine can be used to instruct the radiographer to rotate the image clockwise or anti-clockwise until the correct orientation has been achieved. The third step ('A') requires the anaesthetist to temporarily stop ventilation (**A**pnoea). Finally, the last step ('X') is to proceed to **X**-ray. Once the IOC has been completed, the image(s) should be saved in the patient's electronic medical record for medico-legal purposes and maintaining accurate documentation. When reviewing the image, it is important to ensure that the whole biliary tree has been included and that there is passage of contrast into the duodenum (Fig. 4.14). The IOC is considered negative or normal when the presence of filling defects have been excluded. Figure 4.15 demonstrates a patient with metal implants, which can obstruct the view of the biliary tree during IOC. In such cases, the tilt of the operating table or C-arm can be adjusted to obtain clear views of the biliary tree.

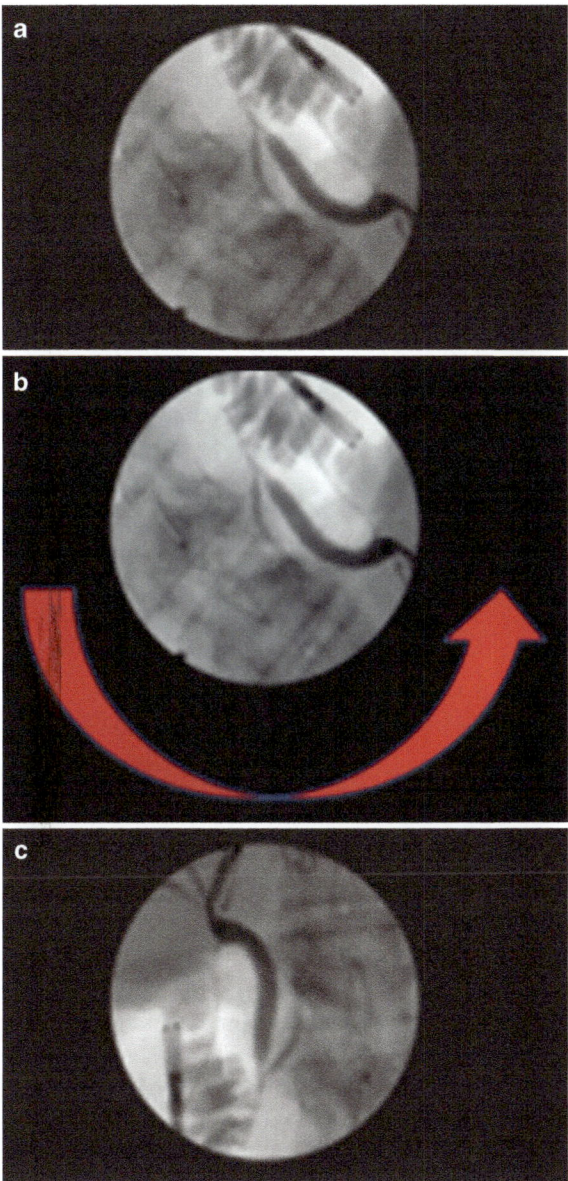

FIGURE 4.13 Orientation during intra-operative cholangiogram (A → B → C)

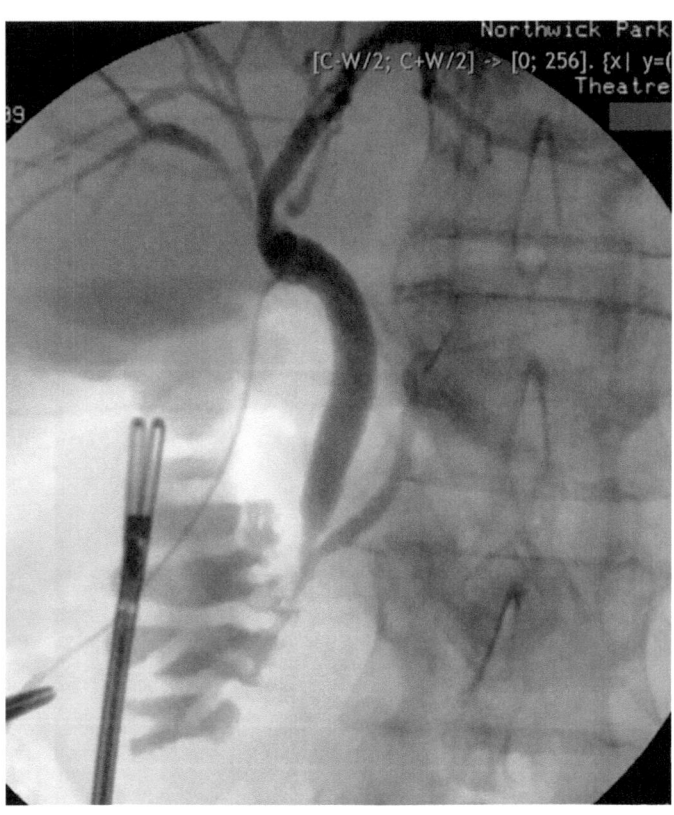

FIGURE 4.14 Intra-operative cholangiogram of the entire biliary tree within view

Not all radiolucent defects represent CBD stones. Filling defects caused by air bubbles are often more rounded, mobile and can change shape. In order to minimise its presence, care should be taken to check the syringe containing contrast to ensure there are no air bubbles that can inadvertently be injected into the biliary tree. More rarely, filling defects can correspond to anatomical artefact. Figure 4.16 displays an IOC with the appearance of a filling defect in the distal CBD in the vicinity of the ampulla (false-positive), caused by a thickened mucosal fold confirmed with 3 mm choledochoscopy.

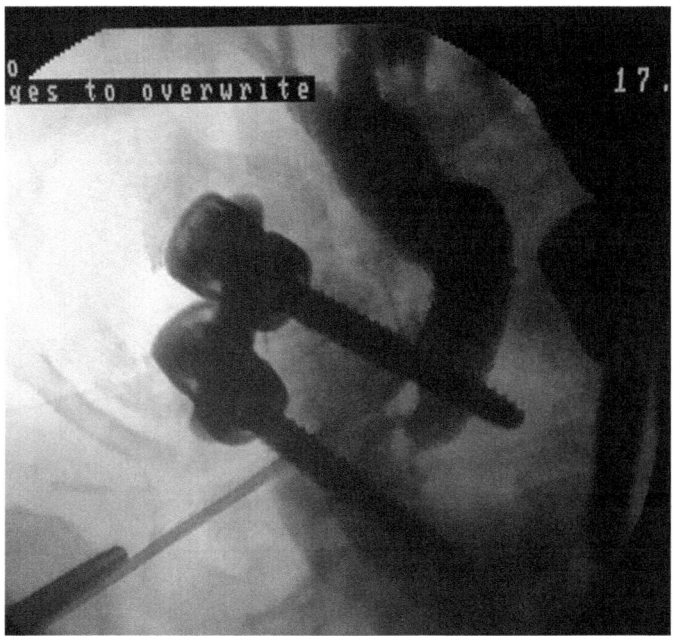

FIGURE 4.15 Metal implants can obstruct the view of the biliary tree during intra-operative cholangiogram

Figure 4.17 demonstrates another false-positive filling defect during IOC caused by a small blood clot, which was confirmed by 3 mm choledochoscopy. In the event of an equivocal IOC, we recommend proceeding to 3 mm transcystic choledochoscopy as this procedure does not add morbidity and is generally simple to perform once the cystic duct has already been cannulated as described previously. If a 3 mm choledochoscope is not available, another less invasive approach that can be used to exclude the presence of small distal stones during an equivocal IOC is the basket-in-catheter (BIC) technique [14]. For the BIC technique, a 5F cholangiogram catheter (Table 4.1, Serial 7) is employed as a working channel and a 2.4F basket is introduced into the duodenum. The basket, whilst in an open configuration, can

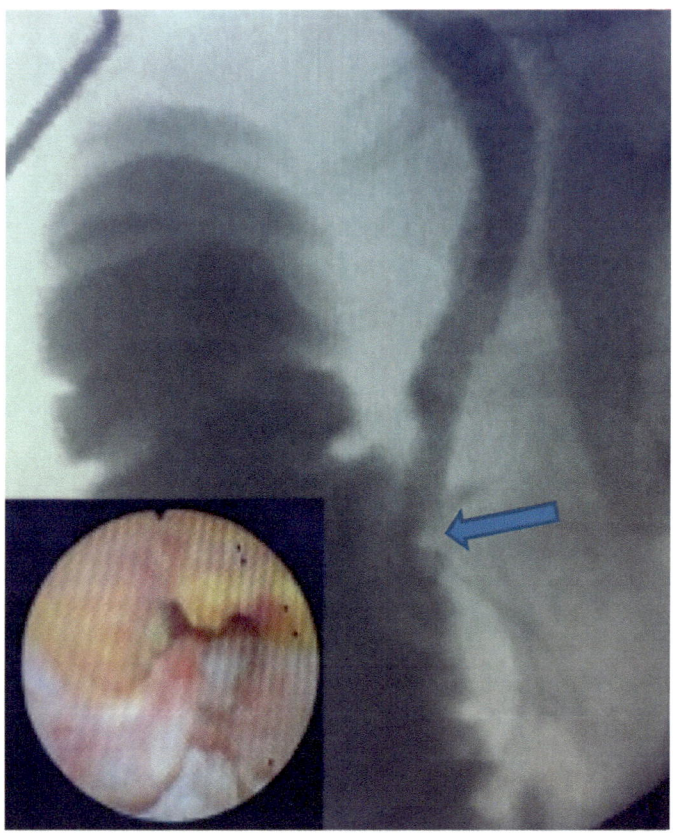

FIGURE 4.16 False-positive intra-operative cholangiogram caused by a thickened mucosal fold confirmed with choledochoscopy (inset)

then be withdrawn thereby trawling the duct. This manoeuvre can be repeated as necessary with or without IOC image guidance.

IOC supported by choledochoscopy can also help to further clarify the anatomy in unusual situations. Figure 4.18 demonstrates a variation in hepatic and cystic duct anatomy (joining duct). The entire biliary tree is filled with contrast from two different ducts, both of which were also communicating with the gallbladder. One was the cystic duct (blue)

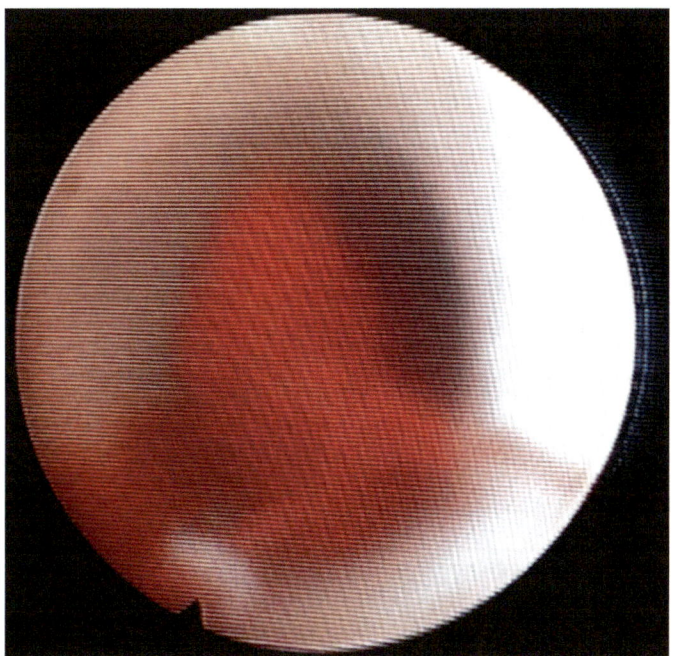

FIGURE 4.17 False-positive intra-operative cholangiogram caused by a blood clot within the common bile duct confirmed with choledo-choscopy

and the other was a joining duct (red) that could have been wrongly classified as double cystic duct; joining ducts are those ducts connecting 2 parts of the biliary tree in this case the duct was connecting the gallbladder with the right posterolateral. Figure 4.19 shows an extrahepatic bifurcation of the common hepatic duct with the cystic duct draining into the right hepatic duct. This anatomical variant did not preclude LBDE via the transcystic route, but certainly would have made impossible the transcystic access to the left hepatic duct. The diameter of the CBD should be known pre-operatively with imaging techniques but can also be measured intra-operatively with IOC and using a ruler (Fig. 4.1b).

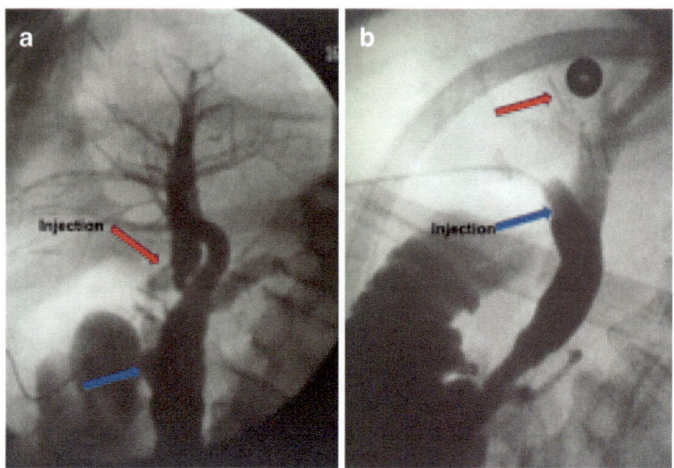

FIGURE 4.18 "Joining ducts"

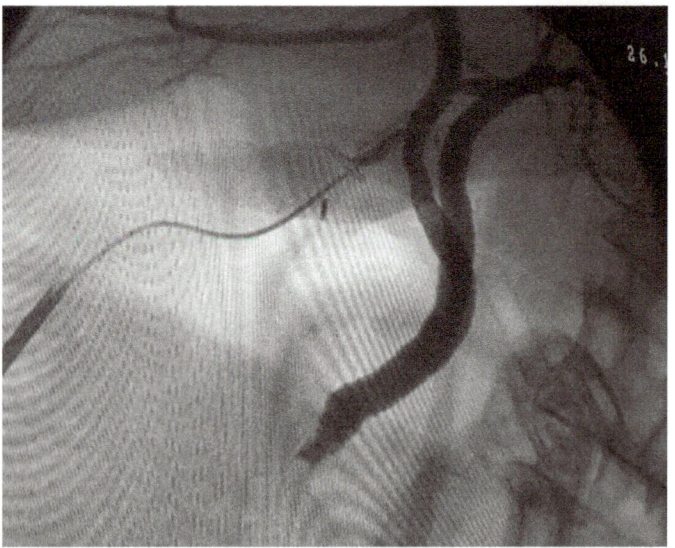

FIGURE 4.19 Cystic duct draining into the right hepatic duct

Choledochoscopy

Once the cholangiogram has been completed and there is an indication for choledochoscopy, the size of the cystic duct needs to be assessed. If the cystic duct is not overtly dilated to allow the passage of the choledochoscope, a PTFE guidewire (Table 4.1, Serial 10) should be introduced through the cholangiogram catheter so its flexible tip lies within the bile duct or duodenum. The catheter can then be removed leaving the guidewire in situ. Next, the 9.5-12F ureteral access sheath (Table 4.1, Serial 6) is railroaded over the guidewire to gently dilate the cystic duct to allow passage of the 3 mm choledochoscope. Ideally the access sheath should approach the CBD at a right angle (perpendicular), but this may not always be possible in patients with a very narrow costal margin, and this will certainly make the cystic duct intubation more challenging. Figure 4.20 demonstrates the insertion of the 9.5-12F access sheath in the subcostal region of the right upper quadrant (left) and the introduction of the 3 mm choledochoscope through the access sheath, accessing the cystic duct at a right angle to the CBD (right). A full description of the surgical technique for choledochoscopy is provided in Chaps. 5 and 6.

When a proximal view of the intra-hepatic ducts is not possible during choledochoscopy (i.e. unable to intubate the common hepatic duct), then a completion cholangiogram is recommended. If this scenario is encountered during difficult cystic duct intubation, then the cholangiogram can be obtained via the choledochoscope prior to its removal, by injecting contrast through its working channel. This avoids removal of the choledochoscope, which is in a satisfactory position, and a challenging re-intubation that may be subsequently required (Fig. 4.21).

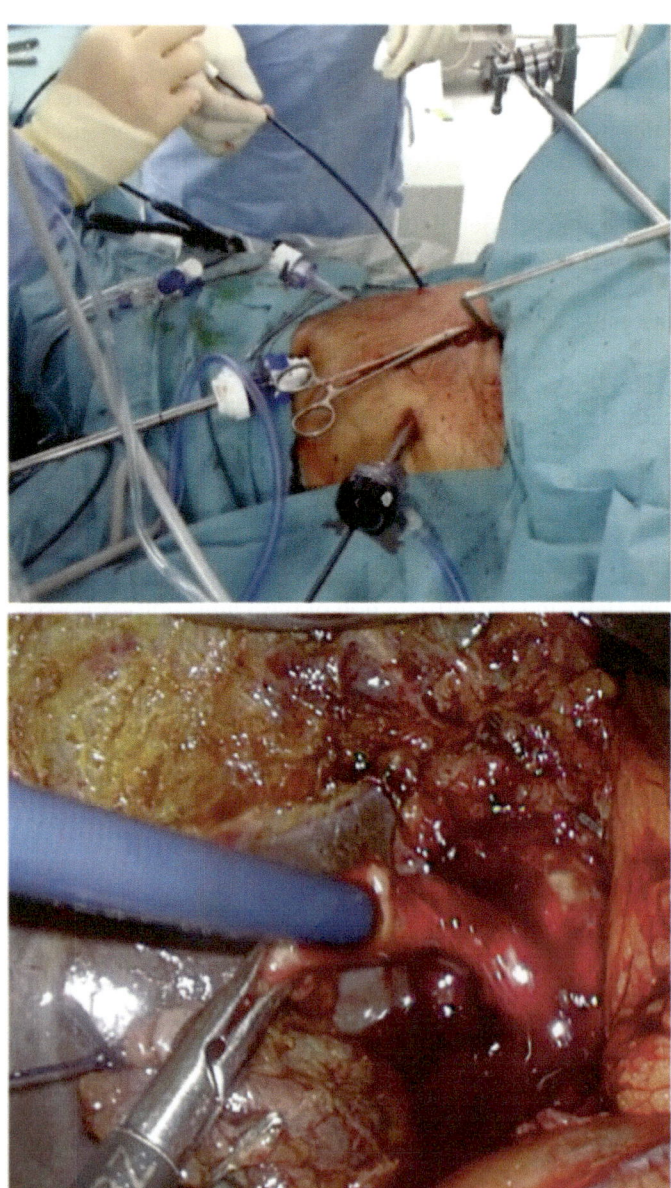

FIGURE 4.20 Transcystic cannulation with 3 mm choledochoscope

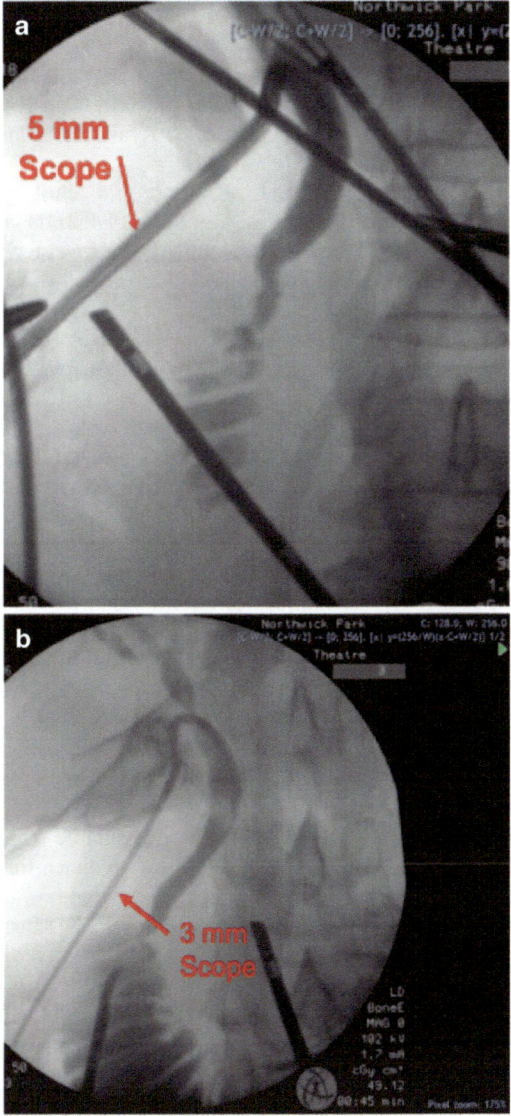

FIGURE 4.21 Transcystic choledochoscopy demonstrated on intra-operative cholangiogram. (**a**) 5 mm choledochoscope. (**b**) 3 mm choledochoscope

References

1. Abbassi-Ghadi N, Menezes N. Seldinger method for intraoperative cholangiography: a practical approach. Ann R Coll Surg Engl [Internet]. 2012;94(4):272−273. Available from: https://europepmc.org/articles/PMC3957509.
2. Dubois F, Icard PBGLH. Coelioscopic cholecystetomy. Preliminary Report of 36 cases. Ann Surg. 1990;211(1):60–2.
3. Marudanayagam R, Sandhu B, Hallissey M. Novel technique of insertion of laparoscopic nathanson liver retractor. Ann R Coll Surg Engl. 2009;91(8):712–3.
4. Yates J, Zabbo A, Pareek G. A comparison of the FREDDY and holmium lasers during ureteroscopic lithotripsy. Lasers Surg Med. 2007;39(8):637–40.
5. Jones T, Al Musawi J, Navaratne L, Martinez-Isla A. Holmium laser lithotripsy improves the rate of successful transcystic laparoscopic common bile duct exploration. Langenbeck's Arch Surg. 2019;404(8):985–92.
6. Martinez-Isla A, Martinez Cecilia D, Vilaça J, Navaratne LNSA. Laser-assisted bile duct exploration using laparoendoscopy LABEL technique, different scenarios and technical details. Epublication Websurg.com [Internet]. 2018;18(03) Available from: http://websurg.com/doi/vd01en5197
7. Navarro-Sánchez A, Ashrafian H, Segura-Sampedro J, Martinez-Isla A. LABEL procedure: laser-assisted bile duct exploration by laparoendoscopy for choledocholithiasis: improving surgical outcomes and reducing technical failure. Surg Endosc. 2017;31(5):2103–8.
8. Consent - GMC Guidelines [Internet]. Available from: https://www.gmc-uk.org/ethical-guidance/ethical-guidance-for-doctors/consent
9. Griniatsos J, Wan A, Ghali S, Bentley M, Martinez-Isla A. Exploracion laparoscopica de la via biliar Experiencia de una unidad especializada. Cirugía Española. 2002;71(6):40–3.
10. Martínez Cecilia D, Valenti-Azcárate V, Qurashi K, Garcia-Agustí A, Marrtinez-isla A. Ventajas de la coledocorrafia laparoscópica sobre el stent. Experiencia tras seis años. Cir Esp. 2008;84(2):78–82.
11. Abellán Morcillo I, Qurashi K, Martinez Isla A, Exploración laparoscópica de la vía biliar, lecciones aprendidas tras más de 200 casos. Cir Esp 2014;92(5):341–47. https://doi.org/10.1016/j.ciresp.2013.02.010.

12. Navaratne L, Al-Musawi J, Acosta-Mérida A, Vilaça J, Martinez-Isla A. Trans-infundibular choledochoscopy: a method for accessing the common bile duct in complex cases. Langenbeck's Arch Surg. 2018;403(6):777–83.
13. Navaratne L, Martinez-Isla A. Transductal versus transcystic laparoscopic common bile duct exploration: an institutional review of over four hundred cases. Surg Endosc. 2020;
14. Qandeel H, Zino S, Hanif Z, Nassar MK, Nassar AHM. Basket-in-catheter access for transcystic laparoscopic bile duct exploration: technique and results. Surg Endosc. 2016;30:1958–64.

Chapter 5
Lithotripsy Assisted Bile Duct Exploration by Laparoendoscopy (LABEL)

Lalin Navaratne, David Martinez Cecilia, and Alberto Martinez-Isla

In 2014, we introduced the LABEL technique [1] as "Laser Assisted Bile duct Exploration by Laparoendoscopy," aimed at decreasing failure of CBD clearance for large and/or impacted stones and increasing the transcystic rate of CBD exploration. Since other methods of lithotripsy can be used to achieve this purpose, we now refer to LABEL as "Lithotripsy Assisted Bile duct Exploration by Laparoendoscopy."

L. Navaratne (✉) · A. Martinez-Isla
Northwick Park and St Mark's Hospitals, London North West University Healthcare NHS Trust, London, UK
e-mail: lalin.navaratne@doctors.org.uk; a.isla@imperial.ac.uk

D. Martinez Cecilia
Hospital Universitario de Toledo, Toledo, Spain

© The Author(s), under exclusive license to Springer Nature Switzerland AG 2022
A. Martinez-Isla, L. Navaratne (eds.), *Laparoscopic Common Bile Duct Exploration*, In Clinical Practice,
https://doi.org/10.1007/978-3-030-93203-9_5

Modes of Lithotripsy

Laser lithotripsy was first described by Orii et al. in 1981 when a Neodymium-doped yttrium aluminium garnet (Nd:YAG) laser was successfully used with a choledochoscope during open surgery to fragment stones in two patients [2]. However, the Nd:YAG laser was less effective on cholesterol stones, tending to drill rather than fragment, limiting its use to pigment stones. Safety issues surrounding the use of Nd:YAG within the bile duct causing thermal injury and damage to bile duct mucosa fuelled the search for alternative energy sources. The pulsed-dye laser converts light energy into acoustic energy, creating shock waves which results in fragmentation of CBD stones [3]. Of the pulsed-dye lasers, the 504-nm coumarin laser was utilised the most. However, there were still concerns over damage to the mucosa of the biliary tree with the possibility of subsequent perforation and bile leak [4]. Pulsed-dye laser lithotripsy has been used via multiple routes to the CBD: (1) T-tube choledochoscopy [5], (2) percutaneous transhepatic choledochoscopy [6, 7] and (3) cystic duct (transcystic) [8–10]. However, pulsed-dye laser fell from favour because of high costs and the limited range of applications, and subsequently laser lithotripsy appeared to fall from vogue altogether for the next decade or so.

Technical progresses have brought the holmium: YAG (Ho:YAG) laser to the forefront among the modalities of stone fragmentation to treat ureteric calculi. In the case of flexible percutaneous nephrolithotomy, the Ho: YAG laser has become the elective intracorporeal lithotripter, being the most efficient lithotripsy method for all types of stones, regardless of their location. Holmium laser lithotripsy (HLL) offered an alternative method to fragment the larger and more refractory biliary calculi with good success. HLL can deliver high energy to a distant target along flexible fibres of narrow diameter. The laser emits energy in pulses, which creates extreme temperatures at the fibre tip for a fraction of time. This converts material into gas (vaporisation) at high speed. Water expands explosively as a gas bubble, which is known as the cavitation effect [11]. There are multiple effects of HLL, and apart from vaporisation, causes rupture of cell membranes and coagulation in the immediate proximity of the cavitation when directed on cell tissue. When directed to solid material, such as biliary calculi, the effect is vaporisation. Furthermore, the resulting shockwave also causes erosion by shearing and contrecoup forces. The diameter of the cavitation is just 0.4 mm, which is ideal for the narrow confines of the bile duct, minimising the risk of damage to the surrounding mucosa and therefore avoiding subsequent scarring and stricture formation. The advantages of Ho: YAG laser when compared to pulsed-dye laser include its greater energy absorption by water, therefore reducing the risk of accidental damage. Moreover, it is less dependent on stone composition for its fragmentation rate, and the optical fibre is less likely to get damaged during handling and firing. The first use of HLL within the bile duct was via the percutaneous route (percutaneous transhepatic choledochoscopy) in 1998 followed by its use combined with T-tube tract choledochoscopy in 2001 [12, 13]. It was not until a few years later than HLL was combined with a laparoscopic approach during LBDE, and perhaps surprisingly, the first few reported cases were via the transcystic route [14–16].

There are studies that have shown that frequency-doubled double-pulsed neodymium:YAG (FREDDY) laser lithotripsy is efficacious and safe in the management of refractory biliary stones by ERCP and choledochoscopy [17–20]. In 2016, the first series of FREDDY laser lithotripsy combined with LBDE was published which included 24 patients from 2008–2015 [21]. In this series, over a third of patients with impacted CBD stones required laser lithotripsy, all using transductal access via choledochotomy. Compared to Ho: YAG lasers, the FREDDY laser functions through the generation of a plasma bubble. Upon bubble collapse, a mechanical shockwave is generated, causing stone fragmentation without adverse thermal effects [22]. Direct visualisation via choledochoscopy is therefore recommended to minimise the risk of tissue injury from the laser. Owing to increased uptake since 2016, with published studies to date coming exclusively from China, FREDDY laser lithotripsy during LBDE has become the modality with the highest number of reported cases published worldwide (>300 patients).

Electrohydraulic lithotripsy (EHL) was developed in the 1950s as an industrial technique for fragmenting rocks. EHL was first applied medically to the management of bladder stones in 1968, which then led to its widespread use for stones in the bladder, ureter and renal pelvis over the next decade. EHL of human gallstones was investigated using in vitro and animal studies in 1987 [23]. The technique was largely effective and power requirement correlated with mechanical strength of stones, but not with biochemical composition. A trend toward higher power requirement was recorded with larger stones and stones over 2 cm in diameter could not be fragmented. Safety studies indicated that electrohydraulic lithotripsy was safe, provided the probe tip was not in contact with the bile duct wall. The probe is made up of two coaxially insulated electrodes ending at the open tip which acts as a sparking chamber. Each spark lasts approximately 1 microsecond and when discharged in 0.9% saline, vaporises the fluid resulting in high amplitude hydraulic pressure waves of varying wavelength which fragment solid objects in their path. In the in vitro study, duct injury was only seen when the end of the probe was in direct contact with the duct wall, most likely due to thermal injury from the spark itself rather than any effect of the shockwave. EHL was the first lithotripsy modality to be used during LBDE, where two patients successfully underwent EHL via the transcystic route in 1992 [24]. Since then, 13 more studies have reported on the use of EHL during LBDE in over 170 patients.

Table 5.1 summarises the different types of lithotripsy that have been used during LBDE along with the pooled number of cases that have been reported from 1992–2020.

TABLE 5.1 Types of lithotripsy

Type of lithotripsy	Number of cases reported in literature
EHL	172
CPDL	23
HLL	141
Pneumatic	15
PSW	62
FREDDY	305

EHL electrohydraulic lithotripsy, *CPDL* Coumarin (504-nm) pulsed-dye laser, *HLL* holmium laser lithotripsy, *PSW* plasma shock wave, *FREDDY* frequency-doubled double-pulsed neodymium:YAG

What Is the Evidence for Lithotripsy during LBDE?

Between 1992 and 2020, 36 studies including 718 patients have reported the outcomes of lithotripsy during LBDE (Table 5.2) [8–10, 14–16, 21, 24–52]. The aforementioned studies have reported on patients from 13 countries across the world. Figure 5.1 demonstrates the trend of reported cases by year from the inaugural description in 1992. There appeared to be increasing interest within the first 5 years in the early 1990s, which then seemed to wane over the next two decades until more recently where larger case series have been published. Figure 5.2 shows a similar trend in reported cases, but categorised by lithotripsy modality. It is important to note that the usual indication for lithotripsy techniques during LBDE is for difficult (large and/or impacted and/or multiple) CBD stones. From the available data, lithotripsy via the transcystic route has been used in just over half the cases (53%). Furthermore, several studies have shown that lithotripsy increases the transcystic rate of LBDE [27, 41, 45, 50]. The

TABLE 5.2 Systematic review of Lithotripsy assisted bile duct exploration by laparoendoscopy: efficacy

Author	Year	Country	Lithotripsy	n	TC-LABEL	TD-LABEL	Clearance (%)
Arregui	1992	US	EHL	2	2	0	100
Birkett	1992	US	CPDL	1	1	0	100
Carroll	1993	US	CPDL	2	2	0	100
DePaula	1994	Brazil	EHL	5	5	0	100
Stoker	1995	US	CPDL	20	ND	ND	ND
Sheen-Chen	1995	Taiwan	EHL	10	0	10	100
Ido	1996	Japan	EHL	54	54	0	74.1
Gigot	1997	Belgium	EHL	3	ND	ND	100
Craigie	1998	US	EHL	2	2	0	100
Berthou	1998	France	EHL	2	0	2	100
Thompson	2002	UK	EHL	31	ND	ND	ND
Shamamian	2004	US	HLL	2	2	0	100
Lo Menzo	2005	US	EHL	1	0	1	100

Muzio	2008	Italy	HLL	1	1	0	100
Day	2009	UK	HLL	1	1	0	100
Varban	2010	US	HLL	4	4	0	75
Farooq	2010	India	Pneumatic	12	0	12	100
Kelly	2010	UK	EHL	8	0	8	75
Joshi	2010	Nepal	Pneumatic	3	0	3	100
Petersson	2015	Sweden	HLL	8	8	0	87.5
Zhu	2015	China	EHL	29	29	0	ND
Pu	2016	China	PSW	62	0	62	93.5
Jinfeng	2016	China	FREDDY	24	0	24	100
Liu	2016	China	FREDDY	89	89	0	100
Xia	2018	China	HLL	38	38	0	100
Gökçen	2017	Turkey	HLL	1	0	1	100
Quaresima	2017	Italy	EHL	15	5	10	ND

(continued)

TABLE 5.2 (continued)

Author	Year	Country	Lithotripsy	n	TC-LABEL	TD-LABEL	Clearance (%)
Ni	2018	China	HLL	10	0	10	100
Fang	2018	China	FREDDY	74	74	0	100
Nitta	2019	Japan	EHL	1	0	1	100
Zhan	2020	China	EHL	9	0	9	100
Yang, C	2019	China	HLL	35	0	35	94.3
Yang, T	2019	China	FREDDY	42	0	42	100
Jones	2019	UK	HLL	7	0	7	85.7
Li	2020	China	FREDDY	76	0	76	97.4
Navaratne	2020	UK	HLL	34	34	0	100
TOTAL				718	351/664 52.9%	313/664 47.1%	582/623 93.4%

EHL electrohydraulic lithotripsy, *CPDL* Coumarin (504-nm) pulsed-dye laser, *HLL* holmium laser lithotripsy, *PSW* plasma shock wave, *FREDDY* frequency-doubled double-pulsed neodymium:YAG, *ND* not determined

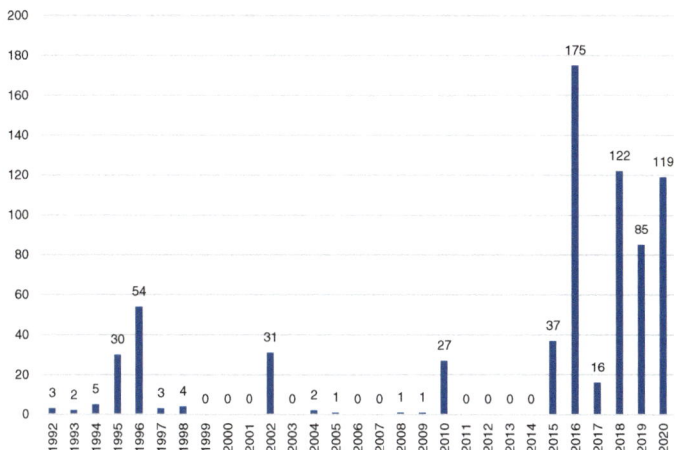

FIGURE 5.1 Total number of LABEL cases published in the literature from 1992 to 2020

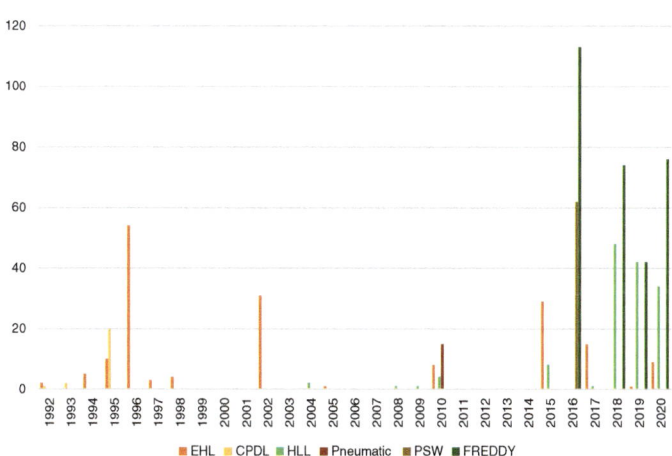

FIGURE 5.2 Total number of LABELS cases published in the literature from 1992 to 2020 categorised by lithotripsy modality

pooled stone clearance rate when lithotripsy has been used as an adjunct to LBDE was 93.4% (Table 5.2). Pooled safety data demonstrates that all modalities of lithotripsy was safe when used under direct vision with video choledochoscopy. The overall lithotripsy related complication rate from 621 patients was 1.1% (Table 5.3). These include haemobilia (n = 2 from EHL and n = 1 from plasma shock wave), retained stone fragments requiring post-operative endo-scopic retrograde cholangiopancreatography (ERCP) (n = 2 from EHL and n = 1 from HLL), and pancreatitis from stone fragments (n = 1 from HLL). Within Europe and USA, the two most commonly used modalities to augment LBDE are

TABLE 5.3 Systematic review of Lithotripsy Assisted Bile duct Exploration by Laparoendoscopy: Safety

Author	Year	Lithotripsy	Lithotripsy related morbidity	Other morbidity
Arregui	1992	EHL	None	None
Birkett	1992	CPDL	None	None
Carroll	1993	CPDL	None	None
DePaula	1994	EHL	Haemobilia after EHL (n = 1; C-D 1–2)	None
Stoker	1995	CPDL	None	ND
Sheen-Chen	1995	EHL	Haemobilia after EHL (n = 1; C-D 1–2)	None
Ido	1996	EHL	None	Hyperamylasaemia (n = 3), hyperbilirubinaemia (n = 1)
Gigot	1997	EHL	ND	ND
Craigie	1998	EHL	None	None
Berthou	1998	EHL	None	ND

TABLE 5.3 (continued)

Author	Year	Lithotripsy	Lithotripsy related morbidity	Other morbidity
Thompson	2002	EHL	None	ND
Shamamian	2004	HLL	None	ND
Lo Menzo	2005	EHL	None	Pulmonary oedema (due to extended op time) (n = 1; C-D 2)
Muzio	2008	HLL	None	None
Day	2009	HLL	None	None
Varban	2010	HLL	Retained stone fragment requiring post-op ERCP (n = 1; C-D 3a)	None
Farooq	2010	Pneumatic	None	None
Kelly	2010	EHL	Retained stone fragments requiring post-op ERCP (n = 2; C-D 3a)	None
Joshi	2010	Pneumatic	ND	ND
Petersson	2015	HLL	None	None
Zhu	2015	EHL	ND	ND
Pu	2016	PSW	Haemobilia (n = 1)	Bile leak (n = 1), haemobilia (n = 1), cholangitis (n = 2), intra-abdominal collection (n = 4), worse hepatic insufficiency (n = 4), pleural effusion (n = 2)

(continued)

TABLE 5.3 (continued)

Author	Year	Lithotripsy	Lithotripsy related morbidity	Other morbidity
Jinfeng	2016	FREDDY	None	ND
Liu	2016	FREDDY	None	Post-op infection requiring antibiotics (n = 4; C-D 2)
Xia	2018	HLL	ND	ND
Gökçen	2017	HLL	None	None
Quaresima	2017	EHL	ND	ND
Ni	2018	HLL	Pancreatitis (n = 1; C-D 2)	Pancreatitis (n = 1; C-D 2)
Fang	2018	FREDDY	None	None
Nitta	2019	EHL	None	None
Zhan	2020	EHL	ND	ND
Yang, C	2019	HLL	None	Retained stones (n = 2; C-D 3a)
Yang, T	2019	FREDDY	None	Bile leak (n = 4; C-D 2-3a)
Jones	2019	HLL	None	Retained stone (n = 1; C-D 3a), bile leak (n = 1; C-D 3a), gastrointestinal bleed (n = 1; C-D 2), exacerbation of cardiac failure (n = 1; C-D 2)
Li	2020	FREDDY	None	Retained stone (n = 2; C-D 3a), bile leak (n = 2; C-D 3a), intra-abdominal collection (n = 1; C-D 3a), CBD stricture (n = 1; C-D 3a)

TABLE 5.3 (continued)

Author	Year	Lithotripsy	Lithotripsy related morbidity	Other morbidity
Navaratne	2020	HLL	None	Bile leak (n = 1; C-D 3b), minor complications (n = 4; C-D 1–2)
TOTAL			7/621 1.1%	45/542 8.3%

EHL electrohydraulic lithotripsy, *CPDL* Coumarin (504-nm) pulsed-dye laser, *HLL* holmium laser lithotripsy, *PSW* plasma shock wave, *FREDDY* frequency-doubled double-pulsed neodymium:YAG, *ND* not determined, *C-D* Clavien-Dindo

EHL and HLL. Table 5.4 summarises the main differences between EHL and HLL. Three studies reporting on EHL did not include efficacy data for patients that specifically required lithotripsy [31, 38, 43], however, from the remaining studies (97 patients) the pooled stone clearance rate of EHL was 84%. By comparison, HLL has a pooled stone clearance rate of 96%. Lithotripsy related morbidity were similar between the two modalities (3% and 2% respectively).

Which Patients Might Require LABEL?

In 2017, our group published the LABEL (Laser-Assisted Bile duct Exploration by Laparoendoscopy) technique for treating difficult common bile duct (CBD) stones and reducing technical failure [1]. Since then, we have demonstrated that use of lithotripsy techniques has increased our rate of successful transcystic LBDE from 67% to over 83% and only one reported failure of stone clearance in the last ~250 patients [50]. Therefore, without lithotripsy, we estimate that transcystic exploration is limited to around 60–70%, which is an opinion shared by other authors [53–55]. Since the LABEL technique is applicable to all forms of lithotripsy

TABLE 5.4 Electrohydraulic lithotripsy versus holmium laser lithotripsy

	EHL	HLL
Mechanism		
Fragmentation	Vaporises normal saline resulting in high amplitude hydraulic pressure waves of varying wavelength which fragment stones	The laser emits energy in pulses, which creates extreme temperatures at the fibre tip for a fraction of time. This converts material into gas (vaporisation) at high speed. Water expands explosively as a gas bubble, which is known as the cavitation effect
Equipment related		
Probe size	800 μm	200 μm
Price per unit	£350	£350
Number of shots	1500	Unlimited
Availability of generator	~3% of UK hospitals[a]	Most hospitals
Special license required	NO	YES
Special theatre required	NO	YES
Goggles required	NO	YES
Interference with video image	YES	NO
Target diode light	NO	YES

TABLE 5.4 (continued)

	EHL	HLL
Efficacy[b]		
Stone clearance	81/97 (84%)	136/141 (96%)
Safety[b]		
Lithotripsy related morbidity	4/116 (3%)	2/103 (2%)
Haemobilia	2/116 (2%)	
Retained stone fragments	2/116 (2%)	1/103 (1%)
Pancreatitis		1/103 (1%)

EHL electrohydraulic lithotripsy, *HLL* holmium laser lithotripsy
[a]Estimated in March 2021
[b]From pooled data

(not just laser), the term has been changed to Lithotripsy-Assisted Bile duct Exploration by Laparoendoscopy, and we recently published the ABCdE (age, bilirubin, CBD diameter, ERCP) score for PREdicting Lithotripsy Assistance during transcystic Bile duct Exploration by Laparoendoscopy (PRE-LABEL) [52]. We found that when using the transcystic approach to the bile duct, the chance of encountering difficult CBD stones (large and/or multiple and/or impacted) was nearly one-fifth of cases (18.1%). The addition of a lithotripsy procedure to standard retrieval techniques increases cost, operative time and requires additionally trained theatre staff. Furthermore, there are often operating room restrictions when using lasers. The ability to predict which patients might require lithotripsy in addition to standard retrieval techniques, by using standard pre-operative investigations, would therefore be useful in operative planning. The consequence of failing to clear the bile duct of stones using the transcystic route is to subject the patient to choledochotomy, with increased bile leak rate, other morbidity and length of hospital stay, and/or a post-operative endoscopic retrograde cholangiopancreatography (ERCP) [56]. Predicting the requirement for advanced extraction techniques, such as lithotripsy, identifies patients at risk of transcystic failure and prepares the surgical team for a complex procedure.

A simple scoring system for predicting CBD stones in patients with gallstones has been described [57]. Several other studies have evaluated various predictors of CBD stones prior to cholecystectomy [58–61]. In 2020, we published a scoring system for predicting the need for lithotripsy during transcystic LBDE (ABCdE Score) [52]. The primary aim of that study was to investigate clinical variables for PREdicting Lithotripsy Assistance during transcystic Bile duct Exploration by Laparoendoscopy (PRE-LABEL). The ABCdE score is composed of four independent predictors of requiring lithotripsy assistance during transcystic LBDE (Table 5.5). The hazard ratios of such factors allowed for weighting of the score: age ≤40 years (1 point), bilirubin > two-times upper limit of normal (1 point), CBD diameter ≥10 mm (1 point), ERCP (pre-operative) failed stone extraction (3 points). An ABCdE score ≥2 correlates with a sensitivity, specificity, and accuracy of 71%, 81% and 79% respectively for predicting lithotripsy assistance during transcystic LBDE (Table 5.6). We recommend using such a tool to identify complex choledocholithiasis, which can also be used

TABLE 5.5 ABCdE Score based on age, pre-operative bilirubin and CBD diameter and pre-operative ERCP (patient data from the UK)

	Clinical variable (predictor)	Score
A	Age ≤ 40 years	1
B	Bilirubin > two-times upper limit of normal	1
Cd	CBD diameter ≥ 10 mm	1
E	ERCP (pre-operative) failed stone extraction	3

CBD common bile duct, *ERCP* endoscopic retrograde cholangiopancreatography

TABLE 5.6 ABCdE Score as a screening tool for predicting lithotripsy assistance during bile duct exploration by laparoendoscopy (PRE-LABEL) from UK patient data

ABCdE Score	Sensitivity (%)	Specificity (%)	Accuracy (%)
≥ 1	94	36	46
≥ 2	71	81	79
≥ 3	38	92	82
≥ 4	18	96	82

to triage such patients to centres with high volume and experience in lithotripsy and advanced extraction techniques. We have proposed the concept of LATEST (Leveraging Access to Technology and Enhanced Surgical Technique) in LBDE [62]. Leveraging access to technology includes using thinner and more flexible choledochoscopes, often disposables, combined with fragmentation techniques such as laser or electrohydraulic lithotripsy. Enhanced surgical technique refers to full mobilisation of the gallbladder followed by complete dissection of the cystic duct to the cystic duct-common bile duct junction. The proximal cystic duct is then retracted by an Endoloop (Ethicon, New Brunswick, New Jersey, USA) to the abdominal wall using an Endo Close™ (Covidien, Mansfield, Massachusetts, USA) to create an optimal 90° cystic duct-common bile duct angle [56]. Enhanced surgical technique also refers to the trans-infundibular approach (TIA), which we have previously described, and is indicated when Calot's triangle cannot be safely dissected due to a 'frozen' hepatic hilum secondary to severe inflammation or fibrosis [63]. From the authors institutional data, we found that our transcystic exploration rate during the pre-LATEST era (n = 237) was 12% with a stone clearance rate of 97.9%, whereas during the LATEST era (n = 223), our transcystic rate had increased to 86% with a stone clearance rate of 99.3%. We believe that the concept of LATEST should be adopted by centres aiming to achieve high rates of transcystic LBDE.

Surgical Technique for LABEL

LABEL is a good example of *laparoendoscopy* where laparoscopic and endoscopic (choledochoscopy) techniques work together harmoniously, often also augmented by radiology (image intensifier and laparoscopic ultrasound). For LABEL, access to the lumen of the bile duct through the cystic duct is the preferred route, but sometimes that is not possible and it is necessary to perform a choledochotomy and use the transductal route (see Chap. 6). As previously mentioned, the main indications for LABEL are when CBD stone(s) are larger than the diameter of the cystic duct during transcystic LBDE, or when the stones are impacted and cannot be removed with standard extraction techniques during either transcystic or transductal LBDE. We outline three principles of the LABEL technique: (1) a clear view of the stone must be achieved, (2) the choledochoscope must be positioned to allow a perpendicular angle between the stone surface and the fibre (the newer 4-way steering choledochoscopes e.g., SpyGlass™ Discover from Boston Scientific makes this easier: Fig. 5.3) and (3) targeting must be under direct vision to avoid direct contact with the bile duct mucosa whilst firing.

Passing the Laser Probe Through the Working Channel of the Choledochoscope

Although the fibre used for laser lithotripsy (200 μm) is smaller than the probe used for EHL (800 μm), it is still very rigid and when passed through the working channel of the choledochoscope (~1 mm in diameter) may result in compromised deflection of the scope. This is more frequently experienced when the choledochoscope is directed towards the proximal ducts via the transcystic route which requires a high degree of deflection. Furthermore, there are situations which may require lithotripsy whilst the choledochoscope is in maximal or near maximal deflection. In this scenario, you may experience that the laser fibre doesn't move easily within

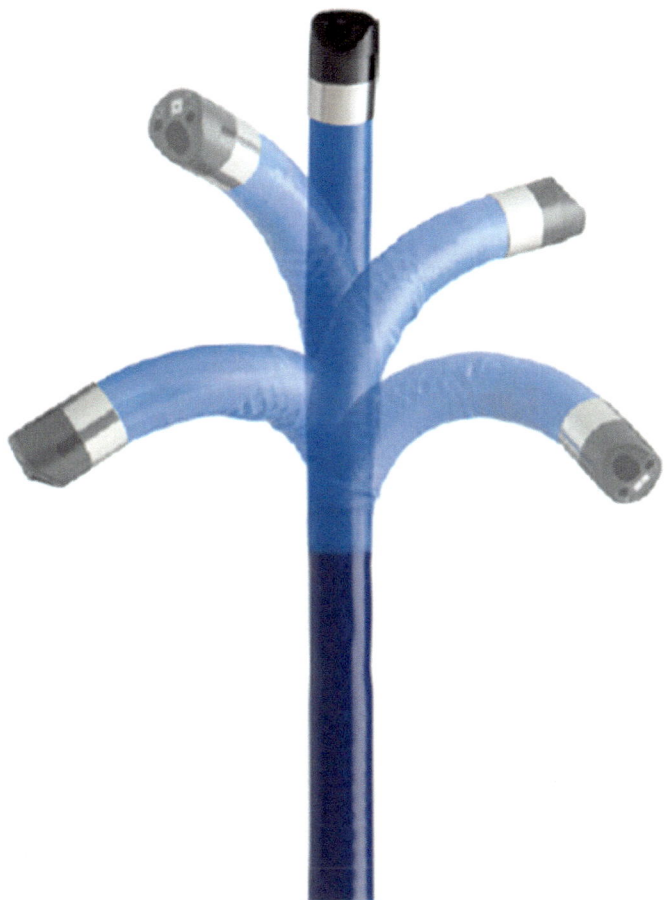

FIGURE 5.3 An example of a 4-way steering choledochoscope (SpyGlass™ Discover) (with permission from Boston Scientific, Marlborough, Massachusetts, USA)

the scope. The work around to this problem is to remove the choledochoscope and straighten the scope. Advance the laser fibre until it is just protruding from the tip of the choledochoscope, then withdraw the fibre so it is flush with the tip of the scope. Re-insert the choledochoscope and despite high degrees of defection, the laser fibre should be able to be advanced enough to be used safely and effectively. An additional reason to try this is because advancing a laser fibre all the way through the working channel whilst the choledocho-scope is fully deflected can (rarely) cause the fibre to perforate through the shaft of a disposable scope.

Aiming at the Stone

At the authors institution, the Ho:YAG laser is preferred because the laser fibre has smaller diameter and a visible diode allows for safe targeting of the stone (Fig. 5.4). This may prevent collateral damage to the bile duct mucosa (Fig. 5.5) [64, 65]. As shown in Fig. 5.4, the targeting diode must be aimed at the stone perpendicular to the stone surface and separate to the bile duct mucosa to avoid iatrogenic injury.

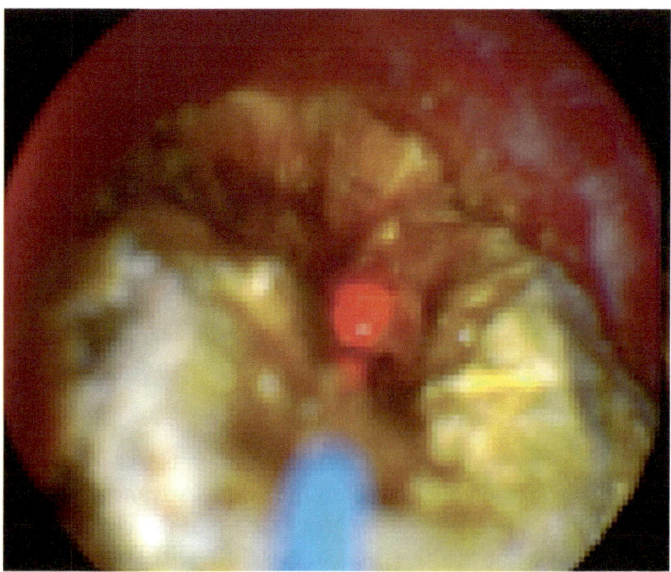

FIGURE 5.4 Holmium laser fibre with visible diode which allows safe targeting of the stone

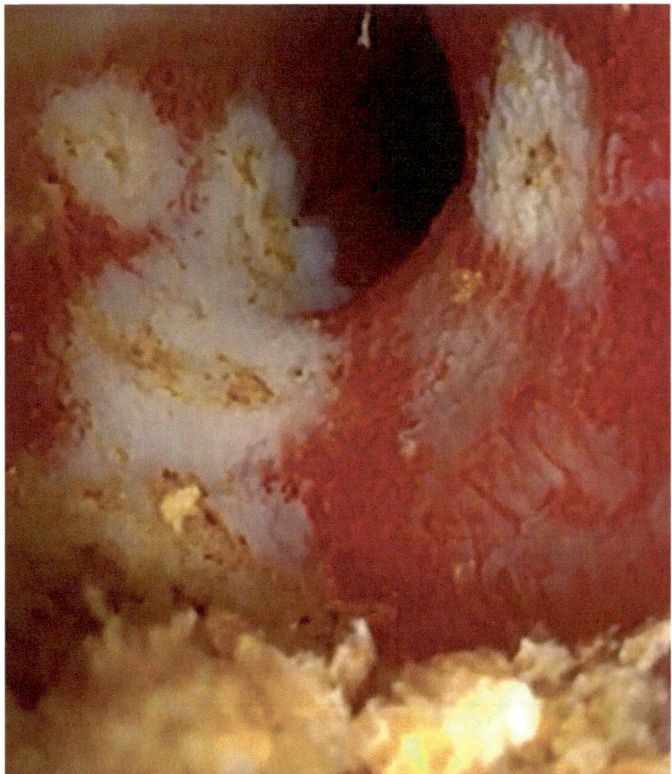

FIGURE 5.5 Collateral damage to the bile duct mucosa

Fragmentation vs Powderization

There are two main parameters determining the action of the laser: the pulse energy (PE) and the frequency (Fr). The PE is measured in Joules (J) and the frequency in Hertz (Hz). Power, in watts (W), is the product of energy and frequency:

$$\text{Power}\left(W\right) = \text{Energy}\left(J\right) \times \text{Frequency}\left(Hz\right)$$

In general terms, increasing the Fr will increase the speed, and therefore also the power. The setting of PE will be influenced by certain factors, namely the stone density and the desired fragment size. The desired fragment size will depend on one of two scenarios: do you want to achieve fragmentation or powderization? Figure 5.6 and Table 5.7 outline these two scenarios. If your patient has had a failed pre-operative ERCP due to an impacted CBD stone, but a sphincterotomy

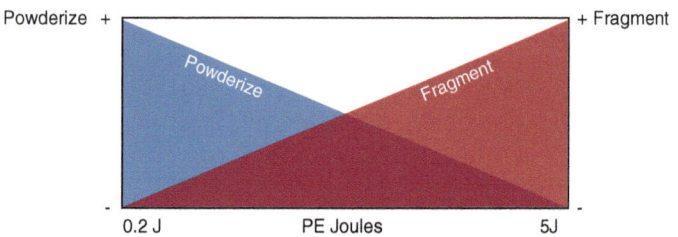

FIGURE 5.6 Fragmentation vs powderization. Increasing the PE will favour fragmentation whereas a lower PE will result in powderization. PE, pulse energy

TABLE 5.7 Fragmentation vs powderization

	Powderization	**Fragmentation**
Previous ERCP + ES	Yes	No
PE setting	Low (~0.2 J)	High (~1 J)
Fr setting	Can be increased to reduce lithotripsy time	Can be increased to reduce lithotripsy time
Clearance of fragments	Irrigation will wash small fragments through the papilla into the duodenum	Extraction with basket
Lithotripsy time	Longer	Shorter
Extraction time	Shorter (or none)	Longer

ERCP endoscopic retrograde cholangiopancreatography, *ES* endoscopic sphincterotomy, *PE* pulse energy, *Fr* frequency

was performed, an appropriate strategy would be to powderize the stone and let the continuous irrigation wash the small fragments into the duodenum. This technique has been previously described as the dusting technique (Fig. 5.7) [66]. A

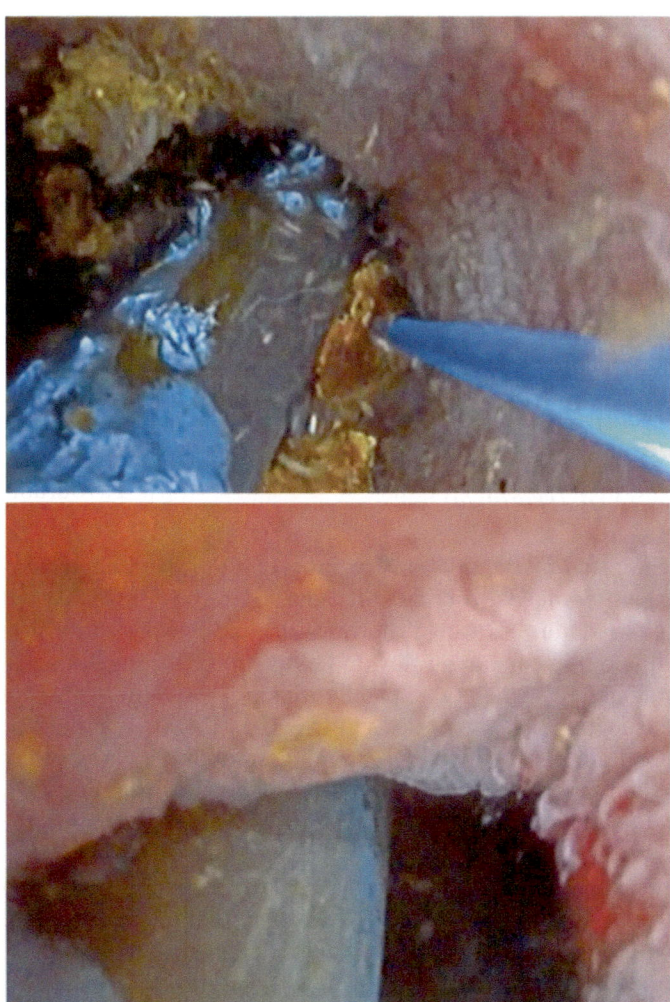

FIGURE 5.7 Dusting technique

lower PE setting of 0.2 J will be required for this approach
and the frequency can be increased to increase the power and
reduce the overall lithotripsy time. The other scenario is when
your patient has not undergone a previous sphincterotomy
and therefore passage of all fragments through the papilla is
unlikely. The resulting fragments will need to be small enough
for basket extraction through the cystic duct (in the majority
of cases) or choledochotomy. For this, the PE should be
increased to 1 J, which is considered a relatively high setting
for lithotripsy and will cause fragmentation (Fig. 5.8). The
dusting technique (powderization) takes longer in terms of
lithotripsy time; however, it is important to remember that
with fragmentation, the extraction time will be longer as individual fragments will need to be removed with a basket. Pre-
operative imaging allows measurement of the size and
density of the stone, which can be used to predict lithotripsy
time and difficulty. Figure 5.9 shows a very large stone with a
high calcium content (bright white on CT) predicting a
lengthy and difficult lithotripsy procedure.

Rate of Irrigation

The rate of irrigation is very important during choledochoscopy and needs to be adapted during the various phases of
the procedure. During lithotripsy (mainly powderization) we
should be keep a high flow to help with the passage of small
fragments through the papilla. Similarly, for lithotripsy of
intrahepatic fragments, a high irrigation flow rate should be
maintained which will help to move stone fragments distally.
When PE is set to fragmentation mode, the irrigation flow
rate should be slowed down after lithotripsy to facilitate the
capture of stone fragments with the basket. Newer choledochoscopes (e.g., Spy Discover DS Direct Visualisation System
from Boston Scientific) have a working channel that can also
be used for aspiration and therefore augment the dual dedicated irrigation channels to achieve a high flow rate (Fig. 5.10).
We recommend the use of a foot pump for irrigation so the

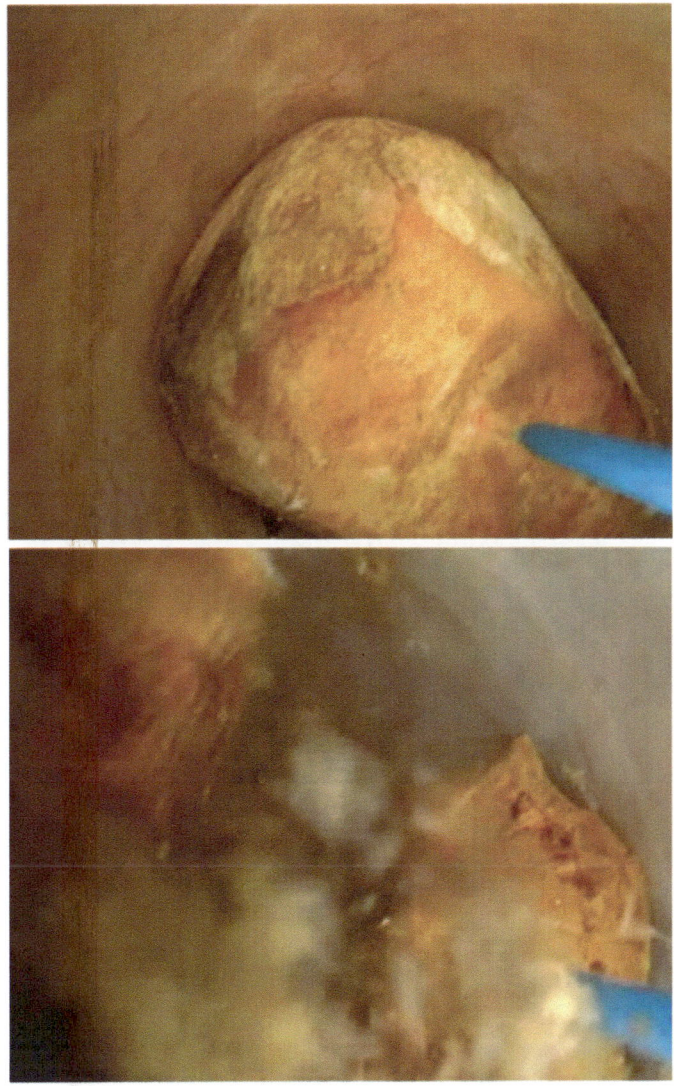

FIGURE 5.8 Fragmentation

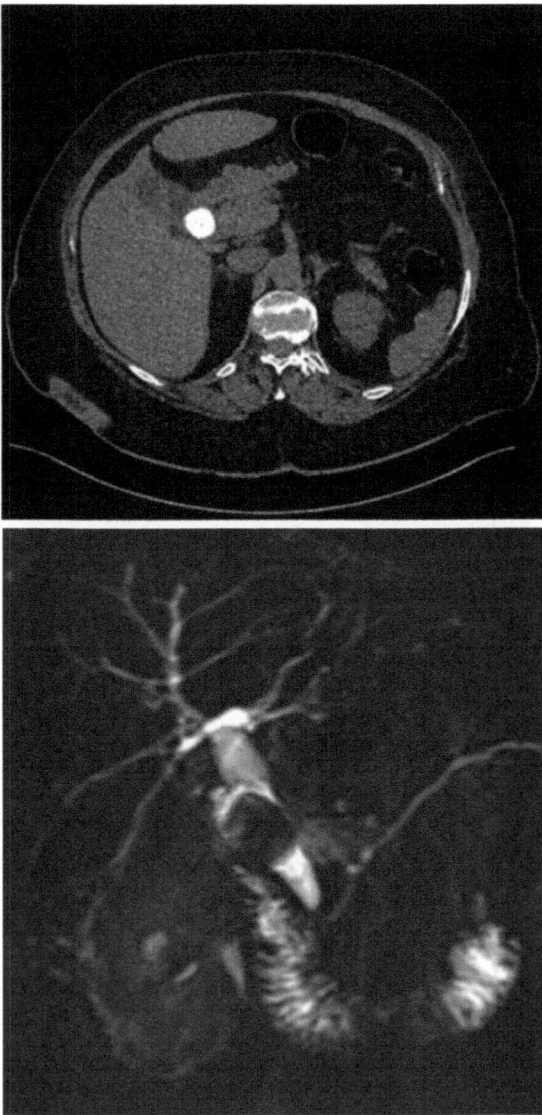

FIGURE 5.9 Pre-operative imaging allows measurement of the size and density of the stone, which can be used to predict lithotripsy time and difficulty

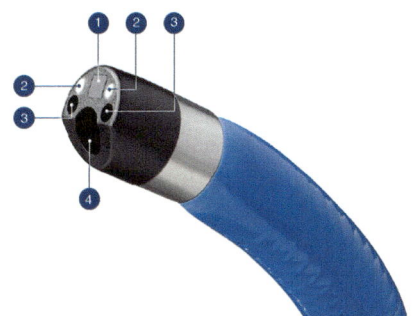

SPYGLASS DISCOVER DISTAL TIP

Equipped for both diagnostic
and therapeutic procedures,
the tip consists of:

① CMOS VIDEO IMAGING SENSOR

**② INTEGRATED DUAL
LED LIGHT SOURCE**

**③ DUAL DEDICATED
IRRIGATION CHANNELS**

**④ 1.2MM WORKING CHANNEL FOR
ACCESSORIES AND ASPIRATION**

FIGURE 5.10 SpyGlass™ Discover with dual irrigation and 1.2 mm working channels by Boston Scientific (with permission from Boston Scientific, Marlborough, Massachusetts, USA)

operator can control the flow rate. Furthermore, the traditional use of saline bags is time consuming for the nursing staff and offers poor control of the irrigation flow rate. High flow irrigation will also help to prevent thermal injuries that may happen when the laser is used for long periods at high power settings (>40 W).

Damage to the Laser Fibre

During lengthy lithotripsies, the fibre tip may get damaged (fibre tip degradation) or bent. In such cases, after setting the laser device on standby and removing the laser fibre, it may be worth trying to cut the damaged tip with scissors and trying again prior to opening a new fibre. As a general rule, the higher PE used, the more likely that the fibre tip will degrade.

Iatrogenic Injury to the Bile Duct Mucosa

Perforation of the ureter is an uncommon but well-known complication experienced by urologists during lithotripsy due to the high volume of procedures that they perform. To date at the authors institution, there has not been a perforation of the bile duct, although superficial mucosal burns have been observed after lateral deflection of energy. In our experience, this has not required any treatment. If a ductal perforation does occur, the CBD should be drained, ideally with a transcystic drain or with a T-tube or anterograde stent if the lithotripsy was performed via the transductal route. Energy and frequency settings will determine the total power in watts (PE (J) × Fr (Hz) = Power (W)). High power settings will induce higher temperatures, which can be mitigated with intermittent laser firing and high irrigation rates, which will reduce the power to 20 W. In an experimental porcine model, 40 W were needed for 18 seconds in order to induce thermal injury [67]. From our experience, with the standard settings, it is difficult to achieve power readings as high as 40 W.

References

1. Navarro-Sánchez A, Ashrafian H, Segura-Sampedro JJ, Martrinez-Isla A. LABEL procedure: laser-assisted bile duct exploration by laparoendoscopy for choledocholithiasis: improving surgical outcomes and reducing technical failure. Surg Endosc. 2017;31(5):2103–2108. https://doi.org/10.1007/s00464-016-5206-1

2. Orii K, Nakahara A, Takase Y, Ozaki A, Sakita T, Iwasaki Y. Choledocholithotomy by Yag laser with a choledochofiberscope: case reports of two patients. Surgery. 1981;90(1):120–2.

3. Murray A, Basu R, Fairclough PD, Wood RF. Gallstone lithotripsy with the pulsed dye laser: in vitro studies. Br J Surg. 1989;76(5):457–60. https://doi.org/10.1002/bjs.1800760511.

4. Spindel ML, Moslem A, Bhatia KS, et al. Comparison of holmium and flashlamp pumped dye lasers for use in lithotripsy of biliary calculi. Lasers Surg Med. 1992;12(5):482–9. https://doi.org/10.1002/lsm.1900120505.

5. Josephs LG, Birkett DH. Laser lithotripsy for the management of retained stones. Arch Surg May 1992;127(5):603–4; discussion 604–5. https://doi.org/10.1001/archsurg.1992.01420050131017.

6. Stoker ME, Vose J, O'Mara P, Maini BS. Laparoscopic cholecystectomy. A clinical and financial analysis of 280 operations.

Arch Surg May 1992;127(5):589–94; discussion 594–5. https://doi.org/10.1001/archsurg.1992.01420050117015.

7. Prat F, Fritsch J, Choury AD, Frouge C, Marteau V, Etienne JP. Laser lithotripsy of difficult biliary stones. Gastrointest Endosc. 1994;40(3):290–5. https://doi.org/10.1016/s0016-5107(94)70058-3.

8. Birkett DH. Technique of cholangiography and cystic-duct choledochoscopy at the time of laparoscopic cholecystectomy for laser lithotripsy. Surg Endosc. 1992;6(5):252–4. https://doi.org/10.1007/BF02498815.

9. Carroll B, Chandra M, Papaioannou T, Daykhovsky L, Grundfest W, Phillips E. Biliary lithotripsy as an adjunct to laparoscopic common bile duct stone extraction. Surg Endosc. 1993;7(4):356–9. https://doi.org/10.1007/bf00725957.

10. Stoker ME. Common bile duct exploration in the era of laparoscopic surgery. Arch Surg. 1995;130(3):265–8; discussion 268–9. doi:https://doi.org/10.1001/archsurg.1995.01430030035005.

11. Schafer SA, Durville FM, Jassemnejad B, Bartels KE, Powell RC. Mechanisms of biliary stone fragmentation using the Ho:YAG laser. IEEE Trans Biomed Eng. 1994;41(3):276–83. https://doi.org/10.1109/10.284946.

12. Das AK, Chiura A, Conlin MJ, Eschelman D, Bagley DH. Treatment of biliary calculi using holmium: yttrium aluminum garnet laser. Gastrointest Endosc. 1998;48(2):207–9. https://doi.org/10.1016/s0016-5107(98)70167-1.

13. Teichman JM, Schwesinger WH, Lackner J, Cossman RM. Holmium: YAG laser lithotripsy for gallstones. A preliminary report. Surg Endosc. Sep 2001;15(9):1034–7. https://doi.org/10.1007/s004640080149.

14. Shamamian P, Grasso M. Management of complex biliary tract calculi with a holmium laser. J Gastrointest Surg. 2004;8(2):191–9. https://doi.org/10.1016/j.gassur.2003.10.007.

15. Muzio S, Cassini P, Martino V, et al. Transcystic videolaparoscopy for choledocholithiasis with holmium: YAG laser lithotripsy. A case report. Chir Ital. 2008;60(1):119–23.

16. Day A, Sayegh ME, Kastner C, Liston T. The use of holmium laser technology for the treatment of refractory common bile duct stones, with a short review of the relevant literature. Surg Innov. 2009;16(2):169–72. https://doi.org/10.1177/1553350609338373.

17. Kim TH, Oh HJ, Choi CS, Yeom DH, Choi SC. Clinical usefulness of transpapillary removal of common bile duct stones by frequency doubled double pulse Nd:YAG laser. World J Gastroenterol. 2008;14(18):2863–6. https://doi.org/10.3748/wjg.14.2863

18. Cho YD, Cheon YK, Moon JH, et al. Clinical role of frequency-doubled double-pulsed yttrium aluminum garnet laser technology for removing difficult bile duct stones (with videos). Gastrointest Endosc. 2009;70(4):684–9. https://doi.org/10.1016/j.gie.2009.03.1170.

19. Liu F, Jin ZD, Zou DW, Li ZS. Efficacy and safety of endoscopic biliary lithotripsy using FREDDY laser with a radiopaque mark under fluoroscopic guidance. Endoscopy. 2011;43(10):918–21. https://doi.org/10.1055/s-0030-1256555.

20. Jiang ZJ, Chen Y, Wang WL, et al. Management hepatolithiasis with operative choledochoscopic FREDDY laser lithotripsy combined with or without hepatectomy. Hepatobiliary Pancreat Dis Int. 2013;12(2):160–4. https://doi.org/10.1016/s1499-3872(13)60026-0.

21. Jinfeng Z, Yin Y, Chi Z, Junye G. Management of impacted common bile duct stones during a laparoscopic procedure: a retrospective cohort study of 377 consecutive patients. Int J Surg. 2016;32:1–5. https://doi.org/10.1016/j.ijsu.2016.06.006.

22. Delvecchio FC, Auge BK, Brizuela RM, Weizer AZ, Zhong P, Preminger GM. In vitro analysis of stone fragmentation ability of the FREDDY laser. J Endourol. 2003;17(3):177–9. https://doi.org/10.1089/089277903321618752.

23. Harrison J, Morris DL, Haynes J, Hitchcock A, Womack C, Wherry DC. Electrohydraulic lithotripsy of gall stones--in vitro and animal studies. Gut. 1987;28(3):267–71. https://doi.org/10.1136/gut.28.3.267.

24. Arregui ME, Davis CJ, Arkush AM, Nagan RF. Laparoscopic cholecystectomy combined with endoscopic sphincterotomy and stone extraction or laparoscopic choledochoscopy and electrohydraulic lithotripsy for management of cholelithiasis with choledocholithiasis. Surg Endosc. 1992;6(1):10–5. https://doi.org/10.1007/BF00591180

25. DePaula AL, Hashiba K, Bafutto M. Laparoscopic management of choledocholithiasis. Surg Endosc. 1994;8(12):1399–403. https://doi.org/10.1007/bf00187344.

26. Sheen-Chen SM, Chou FF. Intraoperative choledochoscopic electrohydraulic lithotripsy for difficulty retrieved impacted common bile duct stones. Arch Surg. 1995;130(4):430–2. https://doi.org/10.1001/archsurg.1995.01430040092020.

27. Ido K, Isoda N, Taniguchi Y, et al. Laparoscopic transcystic cholangioscopic lithotripsy for common bile duct stones during lapa-

roscopic cholecystectomy. Endoscopy. 1996;28(5):431–5. https://doi.org/10.1055/s-2007-1005506.

28. Gigot JF, Navez B, Etienne J, et al. A stratified intraoperative surgical strategy is mandatory during laparoscopic common bile duct exploration for common bile duct stones. Lessons and limits from an initial experience of 92 patients. Surg Endosc. Jul 1997;11(7):722–8. https://doi.org/10.1007/s004649900436.

29. Craigie JE, Adams DB, Byme TK, et al. Endoscopic electro-hydraulic lithotripsy in the management of pancreatobiliary lithiasis. Surg Endosc. 1998;12(5):405–8. https://doi.org/10.1007/s004649900691.

30. Berthou JC, Drouard F, Charbonneau P, Moussalier K. Evaluation of laparoscopic management of common bile duct stones in 220 patients. Surg Endosc. 1998;12(1):16–22. https://doi.org/10.1007/s004649900585.

31. Thompson MH, Tranter SE. All-comers policy for laparoscopic exploration of the common bile duct. Br J Surg. 2002;89(12):1608–12. https://doi.org/10.1046/j.1365-2168.2002.02298.x.

32. Lo Menzo E, Schnall R, Von Rueden D. Lithotripsy in the laparoscopic era. Jsls. 2005;9(3):358–61.

33. Varban O, Assimos D, Passman C, Westcott C. Video. Laparoscopic common bile duct exploration and holmium laser lithotripsy: a novel approach to the management of common bile duct stones. Surg Endosc. Jul 2010;24(7):1759–64. https://doi.org/10.1007/s00464-009-0837-0.

34. Farooq Qadri SJ, Khan M, Khan N. Use of pneumatic lithotripsy for managing difficult CBD calculi. Int J Surg. 2011;9(1):59–62. https://doi.org/10.1016/j.ijsu.2010.08.009.

35. Kelly MD. Results of laparoscopic bile duct exploration via choledochotomy. ANZ J Surg. 2010;80(10):694–8. https://doi.org/10.1111/j.1445-2197.2010.05269.x.

36. Joshi MR. Use of ureterorenoscope as choledochoscope. J Nepal Health Res Counc. 2010;8(2):69–74.

37. Petersson U, Johansen D, Montgomery A. Laparoscopic tran-scystic laser lithotripsy for common bile duct stone clearance. Surg Laparosc Endosc Percutan Tech. 2015;25(1):33–6. https://doi.org/10.1097/SLE.0b013e31829cec5d.

38. Zhu JG, Han W, Guo W, Su W, Bai ZG, Zhang ZT. Learning curve and outcome of laparoscopic transcystic common bile duct exploration for choledocholithiasis. Br J Surg. 2015;102(13):1691–7. https://doi.org/10.1002/bjs.9922.

39. Pu Q, Zhang C, Ren R, et al. Choledochoscopic lithotripsy is a useful adjunct to laparoscopic common bile duct exploration for hepatolithiasis: a cohort study. Am J Surg. 2016;211(6):1058–63. https://doi.org/10.1016/j.amjsurg.2014.01.012.
40. Liu J, Jin L, Zhang Z. Laparoscopic Transcystic treatment biliary calculi by laser lithotripsy. Jsls 2016;20(4). https://doi.org/10.4293/jsls.2016.00068
41. Xia HT, Liu Y, Jiang H, et al. A novel laparoscopic transcystic approach using an ultrathin choledochoscope and holmium laser lithotripsy in the management of cholecystocholedocholithiasis: an appraisal of their safety and efficacy. Am J Surg. 2018;215(4):631–5. https://doi.org/10.1016/j.amjsurg.2017.05.020.
42. Gökçen K, Atabey M, Gökçen P, Gökçe G. Laparoscopy-assisted micropercutaneous choledocholithotripsy with holmium laser in a cholecystectomized patient: an initial report. Wideochir Inne Tech Maloinwazyjne 2017;4:443–7.
43. Quaresima S, Balla A, Guerrieri M, Campagnacci R, Lezoche E, Paganini AM. A 23 year experience with laparoscopic common bile duct exploration. HPB (Oxford). 2017;19(1):29–35. https://doi.org/10.1016/j.hpb.2016.10.011.
44. Ni ZK, Jin HM, Li XW, Li Y, Huang H. Combination of electronic Choledochoscopy and holmium laser lithotripsy for complicated biliary calculus treatment: a new exploration. Surg Laparosc Endosc Percutan Tech. 2018;28(3):e68–73. https://doi.org/10.1097/sle.0000000000000531.
45. Fang L, Wang J, Dai WC, et al. Laparoscopic transcystic common bile duct exploration: surgical indications and procedure strategies. Surg Endosc. 2018;32(12):4742–8. https://doi.org/10.1007/s00464-018-6195-z.
46. Nitta T, Chino Y, Kataoka J, et al. Combination of electrohydraulic lithotripsy and laparoscopy for gallbladder access in type III Mirizzi syndrome. Asian J Endosc Surg. 2019;12(2):227–31. https://doi.org/10.1111/ases.12602.
47. Zhan Z, Han H, Zhao D, et al. Primary closure after laparoscopic common bile duct exploration is feasible for elderly patients: 5-year experience at a single institution. Asian J Surg. 2020;43(1):110–5. https://doi.org/10.1016/j.asjsur.2019.04.009.
48. Yang C, Wang H. Treatment of incarcerated choledocholithiasis with holmium laser in laparoscopic bile duct exploration. Asian J Surg. 2019;42(10):932–4. https://doi.org/10.1016/j.asjsur.2019.06.007.

49. Yang T, Ma Z, Xu B, et al. Clinical role of frequency-doubled double-pulse neodymium YAG laser lithotripsy for removal of difficult biliary stones in laparoscopic common bile duct exploration. ANZ J Surg. 2019;89(9):E358–62. https://doi.org/10.1111/ans.15364.

50. Jones T, Al Musawi J, Navaratne L, Martinez-Isla A. Holmium laser lithotripsy improves the rate of successful transcystic laparoscopic common bile duct exploration. Langenbeck's Arch Surg. 2019;404(8):985–92. https://doi.org/10.1007/s00423-019-01845-3.

51. Li G, Pang Q, Zhai H, et al. SpyGlass-guided laser lithotripsy versus laparoscopic common bile duct exploration for large common bile duct stones: a non-inferiority trial. Surg Endosc. 2020;https://doi.org/10.1007/s00464-020-07862-4.

52. Navaratne L, Martínez Cecilia D, Martínez Isla A. The ABCdE score for PREdicting Lithotripsy Assistance during transcystic bile duct exploration by laparoendoscopy (PRE-LABEL). Surg Endosc. 2020;https://doi.org/10.1007/s00464-020-08082-6

53. Nassar AHM, Ng HJ, Katbeh T, Cannings E. Conventional surgical management of bile duct stones: a service model and outcomes of 1318 laparoscopic explorations. Ann Surg. 2020;Publish Ahead of Print:https://doi.org/10.1097/sla.0000000000004680.

54. Grubnik VV, Tkachenko AI, Ilyashenko VV, Vorotyntseva KO. Laparoscopic common bile duct exploration versus open surgery: comparative prospective randomized trial. Surg Endosc. 2012;26(8):2165–71. https://doi.org/10.1007/s00464-012-2194-7.

55. Narula VK, Fung EC, Overby DW, Richardson W, Stefanidis D, Committee SG. Clinical spotlight review for the management of choledocholithiasis. Surg Endosc. 2020;34(4):1482–91. https://doi.org/10.1007/s00464-020-07462-2.

56. Navaratne L, Martinez IA. Transductal versus transcystic laparoscopic common bile duct exploration: an institutional review of over four hundred cases. Surg Endosc. 2021;35(1):437–48. https://doi.org/10.1007/s00464-020-07522-7.

57. Soltan HM, Kow L, Toouli J. A simple scoring system for predicting bile duct stones in patients with cholelithiasis. J Gastrointest Surg. 2001;5(4):434–7. https://doi.org/10.1016/s1091-255x(01)80073-1.

58. Barkun AN, Barkun JS, Fried GM, et al. Useful predictors of bile duct stones in patients undergoing laparoscopic cholecystectomy. McGill Gallstone Treatment Group. Ann Surg. 1994;220(1):32–9. https://doi.org/10.1097/00000658-199407000-00006.

59. Prat F, Meduri B, Ducot B, Chiche R, Salimbeni-Bartolini R, Pelletier G. Prediction of common bile duct stones by noninvasive tests. Ann Surg. 1999;229(3):362–8. https://doi.org/10.1097/00000658-199903000-00009.

60. Abboud PA, Malet PF, Berlin JA, et al. Predictors of common bile duct stones prior to cholecystectomy: a meta-analysis. Gastrointest Endosc. 1996;44(4):450–5. https://doi.org/10.1016/s0016-5107(96)70098-6.

61. Tse F, Barkun JS, Barkun AN. The elective evaluation of patients with suspected choledocholithiasis undergoing laparoscopic cholecystectomy. Gastrointest Endosc. 2004;60(3):437–48. https://doi.org/10.1016/s0016-5107(04)01457-9.

62. Navaratne L, Al-Musawi J, Isla AM. Comment on conventional surgical management of bile duct stones: a service model and outcomes of 1318 laparoscopic explorations. Ann Surg. 2021;https://doi.org/10.1097/sla.0000000000004951.

63. Navaratne L, Al-Musawi J, Mérida AA, Vilaça J, Isla AM. Transinfundibular choledochoscopy: a method for accessing the common bile duct in complex cases. Langenbeck's Arch Surg. 2018;403(6):777–83. https://doi.org/10.1007/s00423-018-1698-6.

64. Xu G, Wen J, Li Z, et al. A comparative study to analyze the efficacy and safety of flexible ureteroscopy combined with holmium laser lithotripsy for residual calculi after percutaneous nephrolithotripsy. Int J Clin Exp Med. 2015;8(3):4501–7.

65. Nazif OA, Teichman JM, Glickman RD, Welch AJ. Review of laser fibers: a practical guide for urologists. J Endourol. 2004;18(9):818–29. https://doi.org/10.1089/end.2004.18.818.

66. Black KM, Aldoukhi AH, Ghani KR. A users guide to holmium laser lithotripsy settings in the modern era. Front Surg. 2019;6:48. https://doi.org/10.3389/fsurg.2019.00048.

67. Aldoukhi AH, Hall TL, Ghani KR, Maxwell AD, MacConaghy B, Roberts WW. Caliceal fluid temperature during high-power holmium laser lithotripsy in an in vivo porcine model. J Endourol. 2018;32(8):724–9. https://doi.org/10.1089/end.2018.0395.

Chapter 6
Operative Techniques in Laparoscopic Bile Duct Exploration

Lalin Navaratne, María Asunción Acosta-Mérida, and Alberto Martinez-Isla

Different Scenarios in LBDE

Not all patients with common bile duct (CBD) stones will require the same technique for laparoscopic bile duct exploration (LBDE). It will vary according to whether or not the cystic duct and CBD are dilated and also on whether or not there is hilar inflammation (Fig. 6.1). We have found that all patients fall into one of five different scenarios (Table 6.1).

L. Navaratne · A. Martinez-Isla (✉)
Northwick Park and St Mark's Hospitals, London North West University Healthcare NHS Trust, London, UK
e-mail: lalin.navaratne@doctors.org.uk; a.isla@imperial.ac.uk

M. A. Acosta-Mérida
General Surgery Department, Hospital Universitario de Gran Canaria Doctor Negrín,
Las Palmas de Gran Canaria, Las Palmas, Spain

A. Martinez-Isla, L. Navaratne (eds.), *Laparoscopic Common Bile Duct Exploration*, In Clinical Practice,
https://doi.org/10.1007/978-3-030-93203-9_6

153

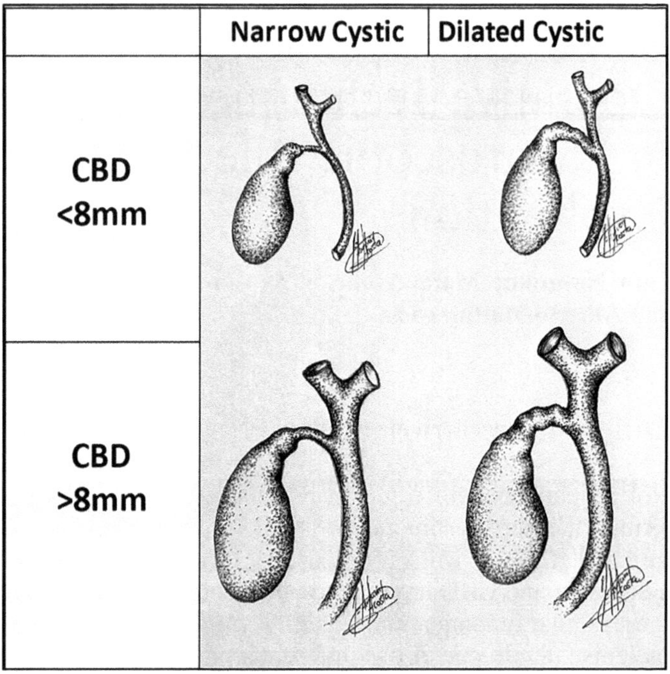

	Narrow Cystic	**Dilated Cystic**
CBD <8mm		
CBD >8mm		

FIGURE 6.1 Different scenarios in LBDE

TABLE 6.1 Different scenarios in LBDE

Scenario	Description
1	Both the cystic duct and CBD are not dilated (most challenging situation)
2	The cystic duct is dilated but the CBD is not dilated
3	The cystic duct is not dilated but the CBD is dilated
4	Both the cystic duct and CBD are dilated
5	There is severe inflammation or fibrosis around the hilum making its dissection hazardous

Scenario 1: Both the Cystic Duct and CBD Are Not Dilated

This scenario will occur when neither the cystic duct nor the CBD are dilated (Fig. 6.2). From the first four scenarios outlined in Table 6.1, it is the most difficult scenario and it will demand a very refined surgical technique; luckily it is the least frequent situation.

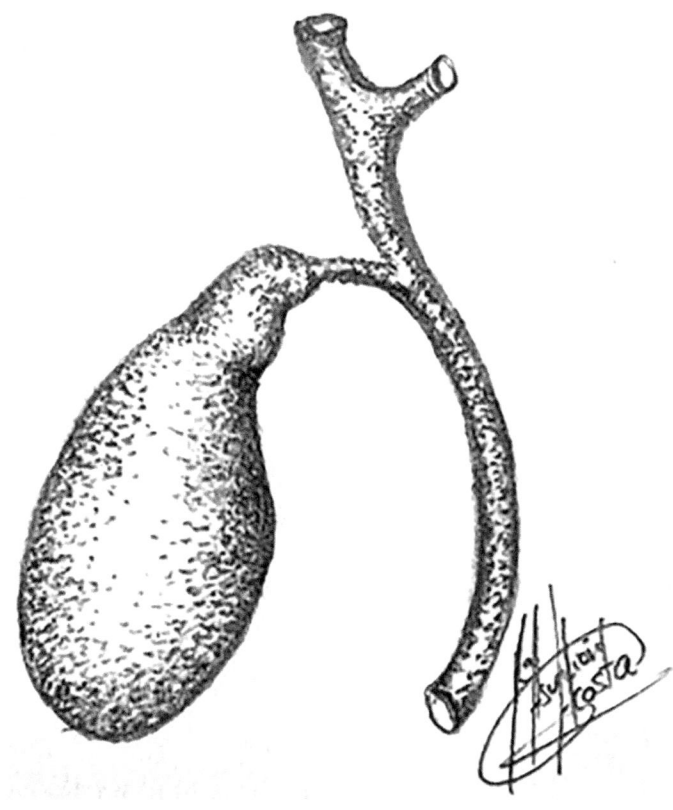

FIGURE 6.2 Both the cystic duct and CBD are not dilated

For the management of this scenario, an ultra-thin 3 mm choledochoscope should ideally be available. The technique described here would typically follow an intra-operative chol-angiogram (IOC) and therefore the 5F cholangiogram cathe-ter would already be in situ (see Chap. 4, sections "Intra-operative cholangiogram (IOC)" and "Intra-operative cholangiogram (IOC)"). The first step is to re-introduce the guidewire through the cholangiogram catheter into the CBD, then remove the catheter. The Flexor® Ureteral Access Sheath 9.5-12F (28 cm) (Cook Medical) is railroaded over the guidewire to gain access to the cystic duct. The hydrophilic tip of the sheath-dilator is soft and therefore will follow the guidewire and pass into the CBD, dilating the cystic duct and overcoming the Heister valves (Fig. 6.3). Once this is achieved, the tip of the access sheath (light blue) is removed and you will need to make sure that the sheath (black) is not advanced too far into the cystic duct thereby abutting the tip of the access sheath against the opposite wall of the CBD at the cystic-common bile duct junction. This will preclude the pas-sage of the choledochoscope into the CBD (Fig. 6.4). If we are using a reusable choledochoscope, we always take great care not to manipulate the scope with the forceps as this will cause

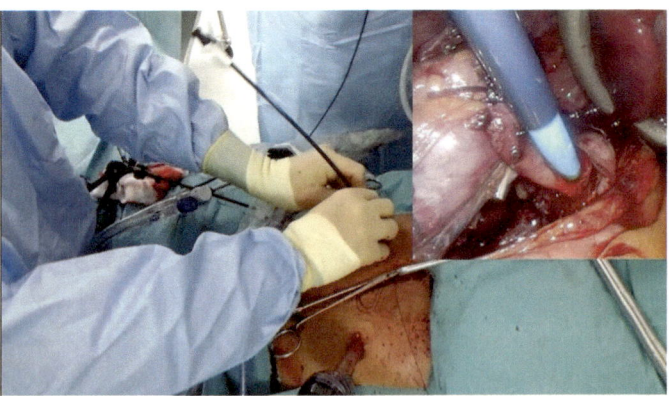

FIGURE 6.3 Cystic duct dilatation with Flexor® Ureteral Access Sheath 9.5-12F (35 cm) (Cook Medical) for 3 mm choledochoscopy

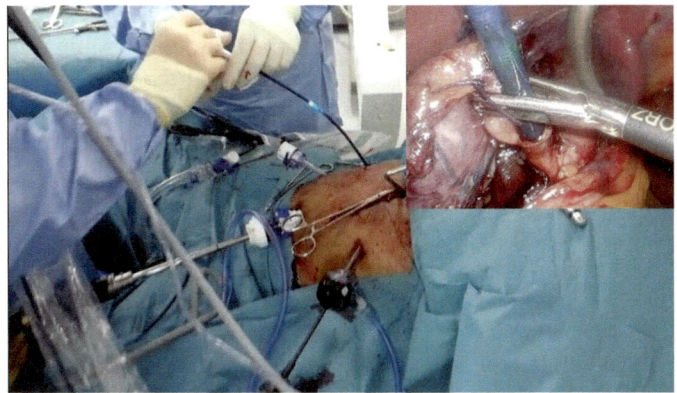

FIGURE 6.4 Three mm scope advancing through the access sheath introduced into the cystic duct

damage and ultimately scope failure. Reusable choledocho-scopes are very expensive and repairs can be very costly which also take several weeks to be returned in working order. Instrumentation to steady the choledochoscope adjacent to the cystic duct entry can be achieved by manipulating the semi-rigid access sheath when the scope is in the CBD (an alternative approach is to pass the choledochoscope through an additional 5 mm laparoscopic port sited in the right upper quadrant). When using 3 mm choledochoscopes, the instrument should be kept as straight as possible because these scopes are fragile which makes it difficult to transmit the torque to the tip. The left hand should control the choledochoscope and the right hand, using the thumb and index finger, will transmit the torque and also direct the access sheath to the cystic duct opening. For this purpose, the access sheath should ideally have a rigid body, and the Flexor® Ureteral Access Sheath 9.5-12F (28 cm) (Cook Medical) works well.

Once the choledochoscope has been introduced into the bile duct, any visualised non-impacted stones can be removed with a stone retrieval basket, of which there are many to choose from. In the authors experience, we prefer to use a 2.4F (120 cm) Dormia basket (Cook Medical) or a 2.4F

(120 cm) Segura Hemisphere™ retrieval basket (Boston Scientific). If a 3 mm choledochoscope is used in combination with laser lithotripsy, we recommend using the 200 μm (smallest) fibre because larger fibres may have a negative impact on the ability of the choledochoscope to fully deflect and therefore successfully navigate the biliary tree. If an ultra-thin 3 mm choledochoscope is not available, and if we face this scenario (both the cystic duct and CBD are not dilated) with a distal filling defect during IOC (Fig. 6.5), we are left with two options. The first option is to dilate the cystic duct to be able to accommodate a 5 mm scope (which is more likely to be available), however, this can be can be dangerous and precipitate a bile duct injury at the junction of the cystic duct and CBD. The second, and safer option, is to employ the basket-in-catheter (BIC) technique as described by Ahmad Nassar and colleagues [1]. This technique involves the introduction of a basket through the 5F cholangiogram catheter, ideally

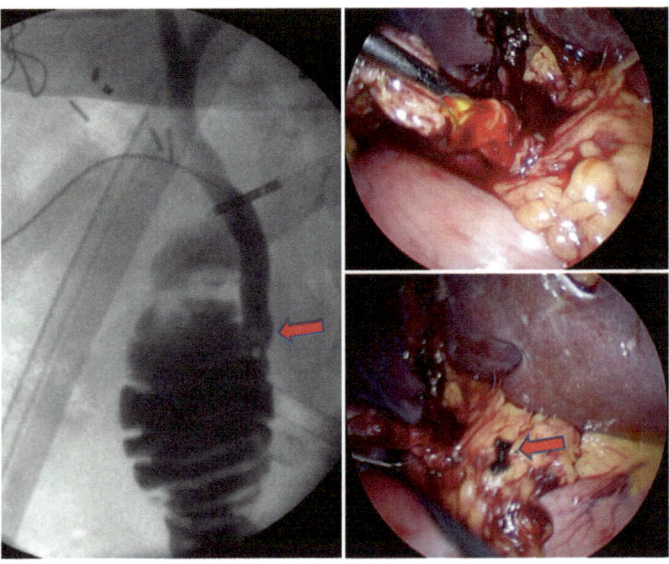

FIGURE 6.5 Basket-in-catheter (BIC) technique for stone extraction (without choledochoscope)

passed into the duodenum, and under fluoroscopic guidance the tip can be advanced beyond the catheter and opened once in the duodenum. Then the 5F catheter and the opened basket are withdrawn thereby trawling the duct and collecting any stones. Retrieval of proximal and/or multiple and/or impacted stones by this method may prove to be very challenging. If the cystic duct can be dilated and this is thought to be the better and/or only option, this must be performed in a controlled and safe manner. To achieve this, we recommend inserting the guidewire (Chap. 4, Table 4.1 Serial 10) into the CBD, then railroad ureteral dilators gradually increasing in size between 6 to 18F (Ureteral Dilator Set, Cook Medical) (Chap. 4, Table 4.1 Serial 9). This should be done gently and gradually as demonstrated in Fig. 6.6. It should be noted that the 18F dilator is the same size as the 5 mm choledochoscope. Cystic duct dilatation can also be performed with a columnar

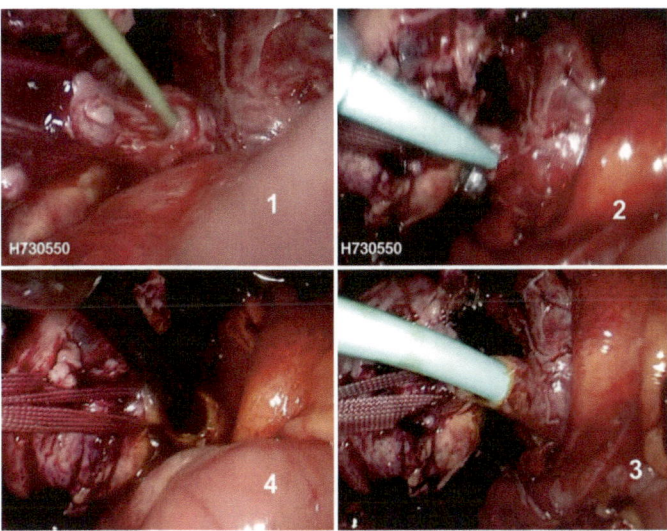

Figure 6.6 Dilatation of the cystic duct in order to accommodate a 5 mm choledochoscope. 1, introducing a guidewire. 2 & 3, progressive dilatation. 4, the cystic duct has been sufficiently dilated to be able to accommodate a 5 mm scope

dilatation balloon; however, the authors have limited experience with this technique [2]. Prior to making a decision to dilate the cystic duct, it is important to recognise the risk of iatrogenic injury to the bile duct, therefore an alternative (bail out) option would be to place a transcystic drain and refer the patient for post-operative endoscopic retrograde cholangiopancreatography (ERCP).

Once all the stones have been extracted from the distal duct (common bile duct) using the choledochoscope, the next step is to assess the proximal ducts (common hepatic duct and intra-hepatic ducts) before completing the procedure. Ideally, this should be done with the choledochoscope, thereby providing direct visualisation of the proximal ducts. To give the choledochoscope a fighting chance of being able to deflect upwards into the proximal ducts, the dissection of the cystic duct-common bile duct junction should ideally be completed as previously described (see Chap. 4, section "Cholecystectomy" and Fig. 4.9). Complete dissection of the cystic duct-common bile duct junction followed by mobilisation of the gallbladder from the liver bed will allow for the correction of the cystic duct-common bile duct angle to a more favourable 90° (Fig. 6.7). The 'windscreen wiper'

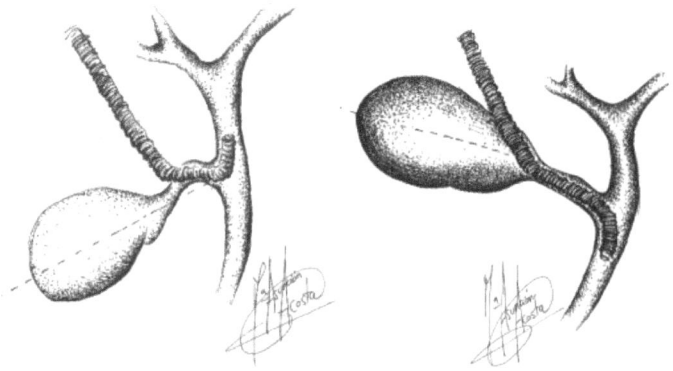

FIGURE 6.7 Complete dissection of the cystic duct-common bile duct junction followed by mobilisation of the gallbladder from the liver bed will allow for the correction of the cystic duct-common bile duct angle to a more favourable 90°

manoeuvre enables the tip of the choledochoscope to move from a distal duct view to a proximal duct view (Fig. 6.8). The manoeuvre begins with the choledochoscope pointing distally, then anti-clockwise torque is applied to the scope using the right thumb and index finger thereby rotating the scope proximally. In the event that proximal choledochoscopy is not possible, a completion cholangiogram should be performed to exclude proximal stones.

There are some situations where transcystic exploration may not be possible. For example, a very low cystic duct insertion into the CBD with a mid-ductal stone may entirely preclude proximal choledochoscopy. Similarly, a proximally facing cystic duct insertion into the CBD, in a double-barrel fashion (which we have experienced only twice), may not permit access to the distal bile duct, and therefore a choledochotomy may be required to achieve distal choledochoscopy. A cystic duct crossing to the other side and draining medially should not be a contraindication if it is dissected properly, however, a thin non-dilated cystic duct may prove to be a very challenging conduit in this scenario [3].

Scenario 2: The Cystic Duct Is Dilated But the CBD Is Not Dilated

The scenario where the cystic duct is dilated and the CBD is not dilated (normal calibre) (Fig. 6.9) is unusual but favourable, because the dilated cystic duct will probably allow the direct transcystic insertion of a 5 mm choledochoscope. Moreover, the stones in a duct that is not dilated should not be too large, and therefore unless they are impacted, would be easy to extract transcystically.

As described in Scenario 1, a similar technique for introduction of the choledochoscope can be used, however, in a cystic duct that is dilated, there is no need for the use of the access sheath. If you are using a 5 mm choledochoscope, this can be introduced from an extra 5 mm laparoscopic port, also inserted in the right upper quadrant. If you are using the

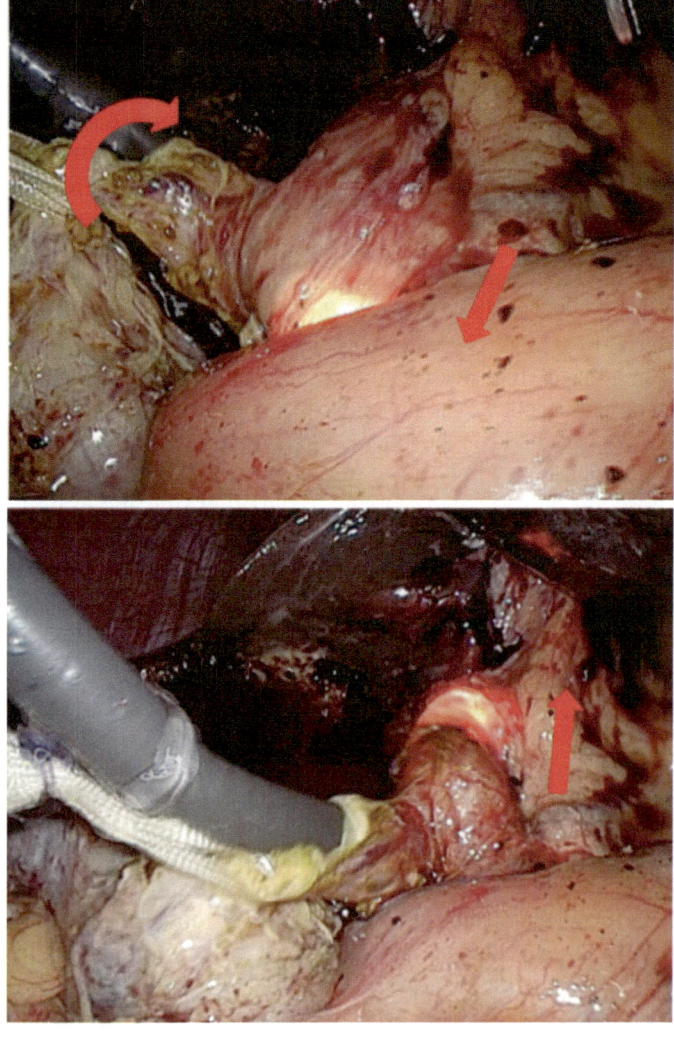

FIGURE 6.8 The 'windscreen wiper' manoeuvre for proximal CBD access

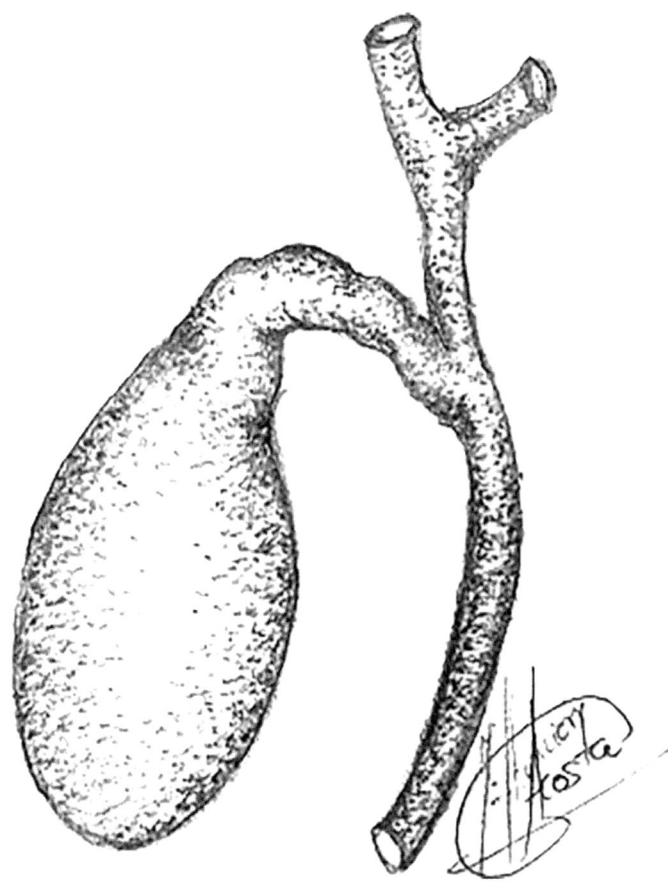

FIGURE 6.9 The cystic duct is dilated but the CBD is not dilated

'American' supine patient position, the mid 5 mm port can be used for choledochoscopic access. The same Endoloop traction technique should be used, but in this scenario, any dilatation of the cystic duct that is required can be achieved using Johan grasping forceps (Fig. 6.10). This manoeuvre will often also overcome any obstructing Heister valves.

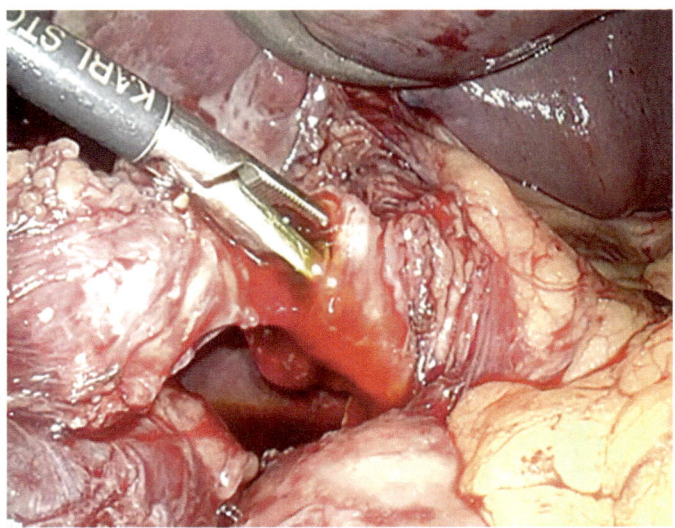

FIGURE 6.10 Cystic duct dilatation using Johan grasping forceps

Scenario 3: The Cystic Duct Is Not Dilated But the CBD Is Dilated

In this scenario, you will find a dilated bile duct with a non-dilated cystic duct (Fig. 6.11). Transcystic access can be achieved using the same technique as described in scenario 1. This should be the first approach, however, if this is not possible, a dilated bile duct will allow for a safe choledochotomy to be performed. The minimal safe diameter of the bile duct when performing a choledochotomy is controversial and has previously been contested. Closure of the bile duct less than 5 mm has been associated with strictures [4]. In general terms, a choledochotomy should not be performed on a bile duct smaller than 7–9 mm [5, 6]. In our practice, we consider a duct as being dilated when it is more than 8 mm.

Generally, large bile ducts harbour large-sized stones, and if the aim is to manage them using a transcystic approach, the Lithotripsy Assisted Bile duct Exploration by Laparoendoscopy (LABEL) technique may be required

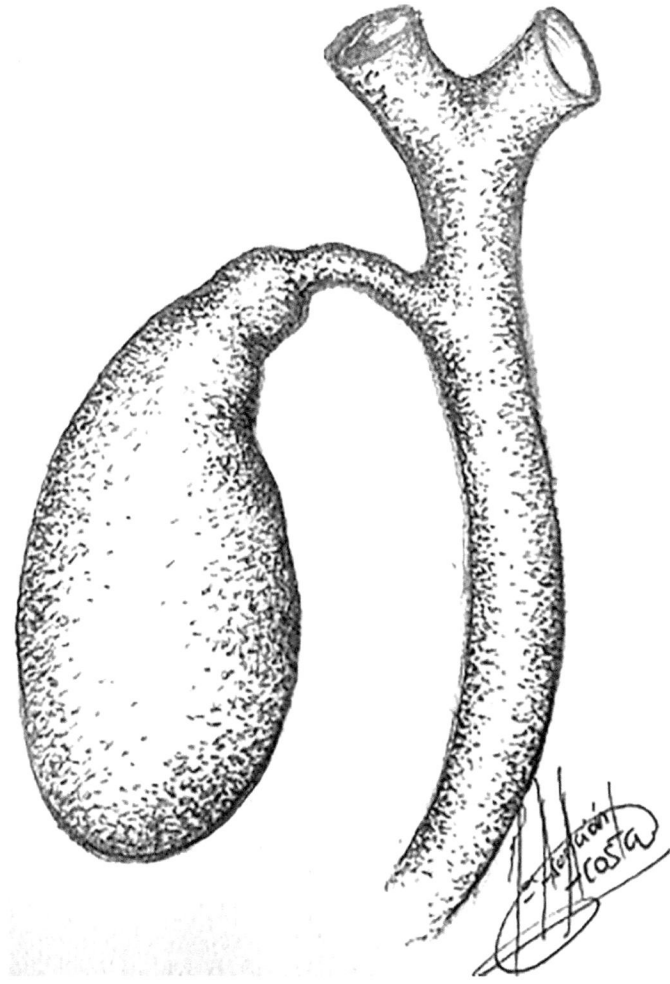

FIGURE 6.11 The cystic duct is not dilated but the CBD is dilated

[7, 8]. In very rare occasions, when the stones are very large and with a high calcium content (best seen on CT imaging), the LABEL technique is used to powderize the stones into smaller fragments. If the patient has had a previous endoscopic spincterotomy (ERCP-ES), these fragments are

powderized and therefore easily washed down into the duo-denum. If there has not been a previous ERCP-ES, and if the fragments cannot be extracted tanscystically, then it may be necessary to complete CBD clearance of these fragments with a post-operative ERCP-ES.

Figure 6.12 demonstrates transcystic extraction of a 10 mm stone through a 5 mm cystic duct. The temptation would be to perform a choledochotomy for easy stone extraction, how-ever, the aim should always be to perform transcystic LBDE where possible. Therefore, in this case we elected to perform lithotripsy (LABEL technique), thereby fragmenting the stone into smaller pieces that are then able to be extracted via the cystic duct using a Dormia basket. It is important to not be too ambitious when extracting large unfragmented stones through the cystic duct. The danger is that if a stone larger than the size of the cystic duct is extracted with a bas-ket, the entire basket-stone complex can get impacted either within the CBD, at the cystic duct-common bile duct junction or the cystic duct itself (Fig. 6.13a). What are your options in this scenario? First, dismount the handle of the basket so that the choledochoscope can be removed. Second, exteriorise the proximal free end of the wire through the abdominal wall close by using a wide bore needle (Fig. 6.13b) or alternatively, leave the free end within the abdomen. Third, re-intubate the cystic duct with the choledochoscope and perform lithotripsy on the impacted basket-stone complex (Fig. 6.13c). Once the basket-stone complex has become disimpacted by fragment-ing the impacted stone, the loose wire can safely be removed along with the stone fragments via the cystic duct opening. However, this situation can be avoided altogether if the stone size is assessed from the outset and the LABEL technique applied prior to extraction of the large stone with a basket.

If the transcystic route is not feasible, proceeding to cho-ledochotomy and transductal stone extraction is an appropri-ate option, taking advantage of the dilated bile duct. This should be performed via a longitudinal (vertical) incision within the supraduodenal portion of the bile duct. In a non-inflamed, thin-walled bile duct, this can be achieved with laparoscopic scissors or a Berci knife® [9] (Fig. 6.14). In a

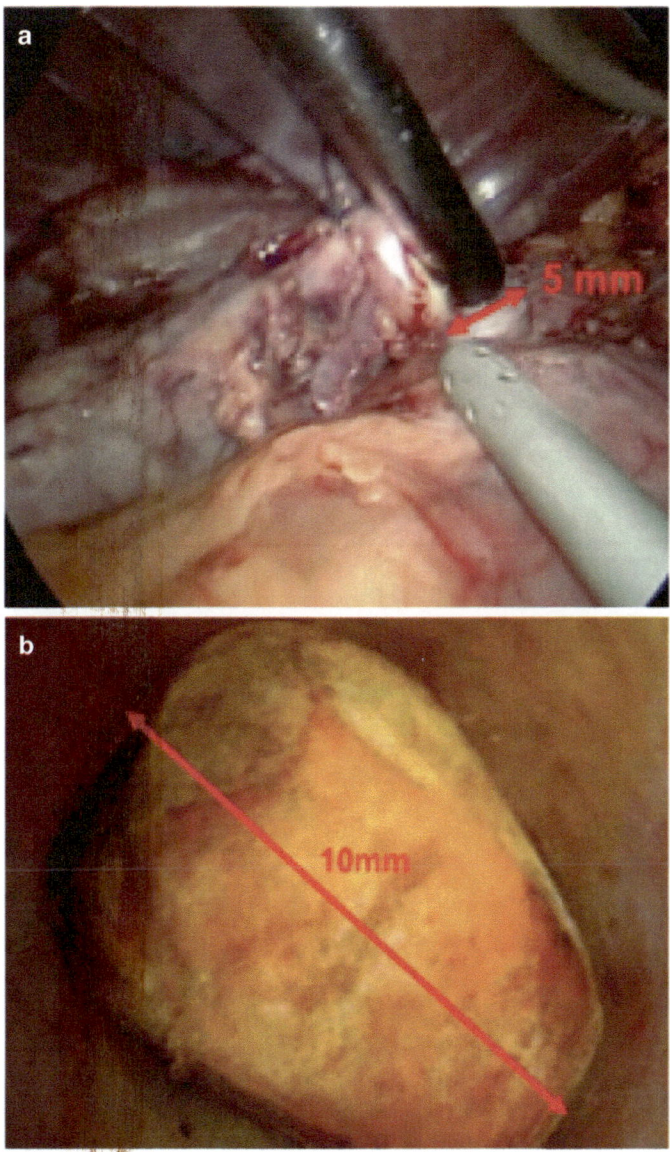

FIGURE 6.12 Transcystic extraction of a large stone. (**a**) transcystic access with 5 mm choledochoscopy. (**b**) 10 mm CBD stone. (**c**) LABEL technique. (**d**) transcystic removal of small fragments

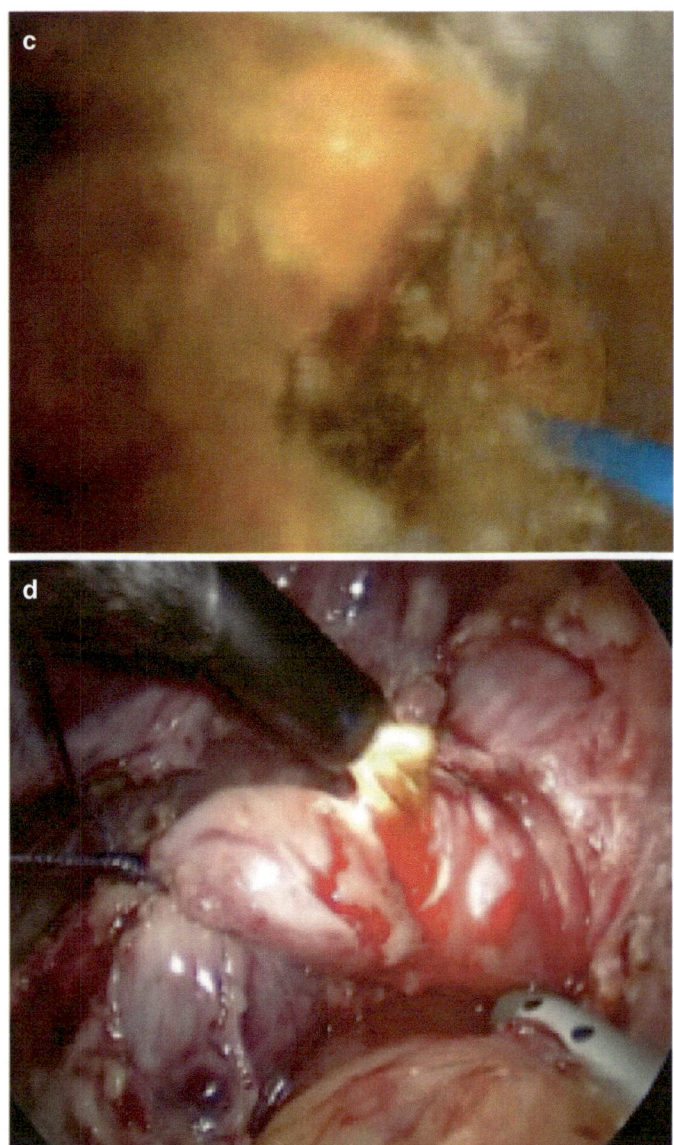

FIGURE 6.12 (continued)

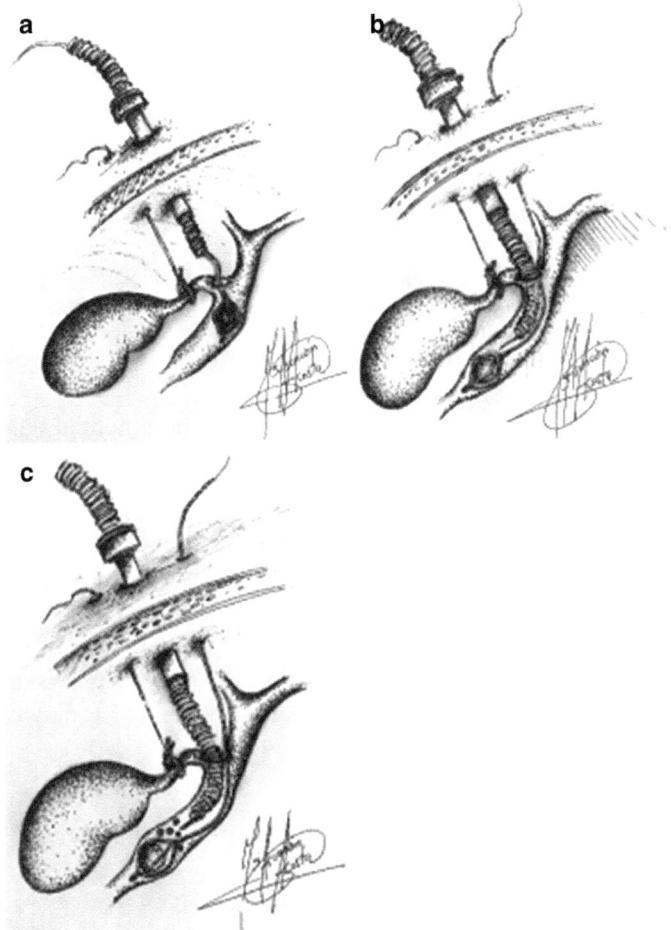

FIGURE 6.13 Impacted basket-stone complex within the bile duct (**a**) and a strategy for getting out of trouble by disconneting the basket handle (**b**) and fragmenting the impacted basket-stone complex using the LABEL technique (**c**)

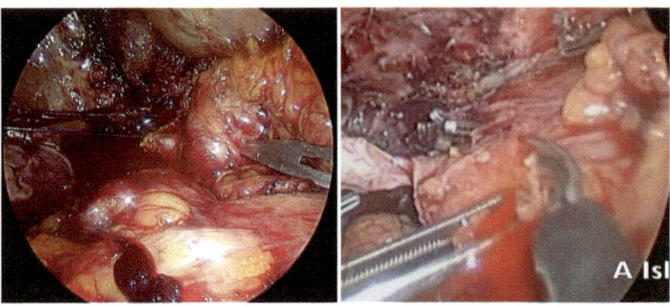

FIGURE 6.14 Choledochotomy incision. Knife choledochotomy (left), scissors choledochotomy (right)

severely inflamed, thick-walled bile duct, the potential danger with scissors or a knife is that cutting into a thickened duct wall can create a false channel and miss the ductal lumen altogether. In such cases, we have controversially used the hook (in pure cut mode) without problems (Fig. 6.15). The size of the choledochotomy should be tailored to the size of the stone. Standard stone extraction techniques include removal with grasping forceps (if the stone is lodged in the mid portion of the duct) (Fig. 6.16) or a Dormia basket. Advanced stone extraction techniques with LABEL may be required for large and/or impacted stones.

Scenario 4: Both the Cystic Duct and CBD Are Dilated

The scenario of a dilated cystic and common bile duct (Fig. 6.17) is an ideal situation, and perfect for the beginner during his or her learning curve. This situation will allow the liberal use of the 3 mm or the 5 mm choledochoscopes for the transcystic route. If a decision is made to adopt the transductal approach, then performing a choledochotomy on a dilated duct should be easy. Less commonly, a massively dilated cystic duct can be difficult to differentiate from a type II Mirizzi syndrome, which can compromise reconstruction of the com-

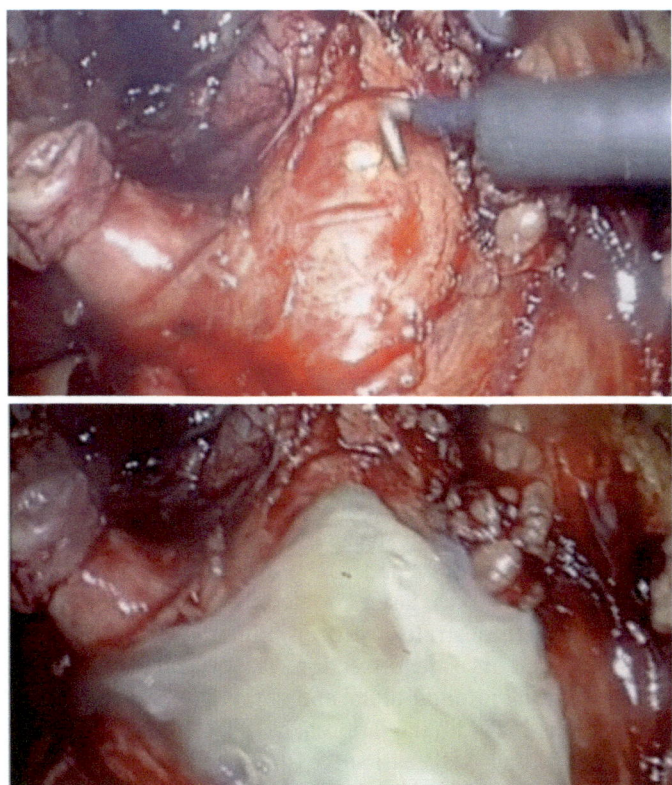

FIGURE 6.15 Hook choledochotomy in acute cholangitis

mon bile duct. This will be discussed next in section "Scenario 5: The Impossible Hilum: Trans-Infundibular Approach (TIA) to the Bile Duct" and in Chap. 7, section "Management of Type II Mirizzi syndrome".

Scenario 5: The Impossible Hilum: Trans-Infundibular Approach (TIA) to the Bile Duct

After several attacks of inflammation, the hilum becomes fibrotic and can become frozen (Fig. 6.18). In this scenario, it

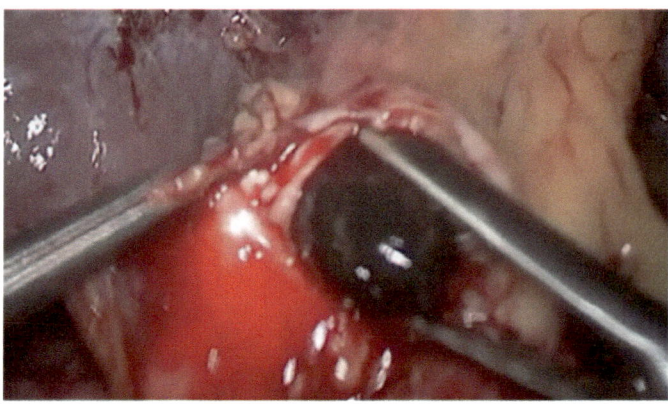

FIGURE 6.16 Transductal extraction of a stone using grasping forceps

is not safe to continue with dissection in order to obtain the critical view of safety. In such cases we have had to resort to novel techniques, often aided by leveraging access to new technologies such as laser or electrohydraulic lithotripsy. Figure 6.19 demonstrates a frozen hilum which was fibrotic and precluded its safe dissection. A very large stone was impacted in the infundibulum, and in this case, we used the so called 'trans-infundibular approach' (TIA) to the bile duct combined with LABEL to successfully access and clear the bile duct. We have described TIA as the approach to the bile duct in cases of a severely inflamed or fibrotic hilum which precludes safe dissection. The inside of the gallbladder infundibulum is used to gain access to the internal opening of the cystic duct and then onwards to the CBD. This technique often needs to be combined with LABEL [10], because in most cases the offending stones are impacted or too large to be removed through the cystic duct [11, 12]. When TIA is indicated, choledochotomy is often also precluded, not only because the duct wall is inflamed and thickened, but also because identification of the bile duct is often not possible.

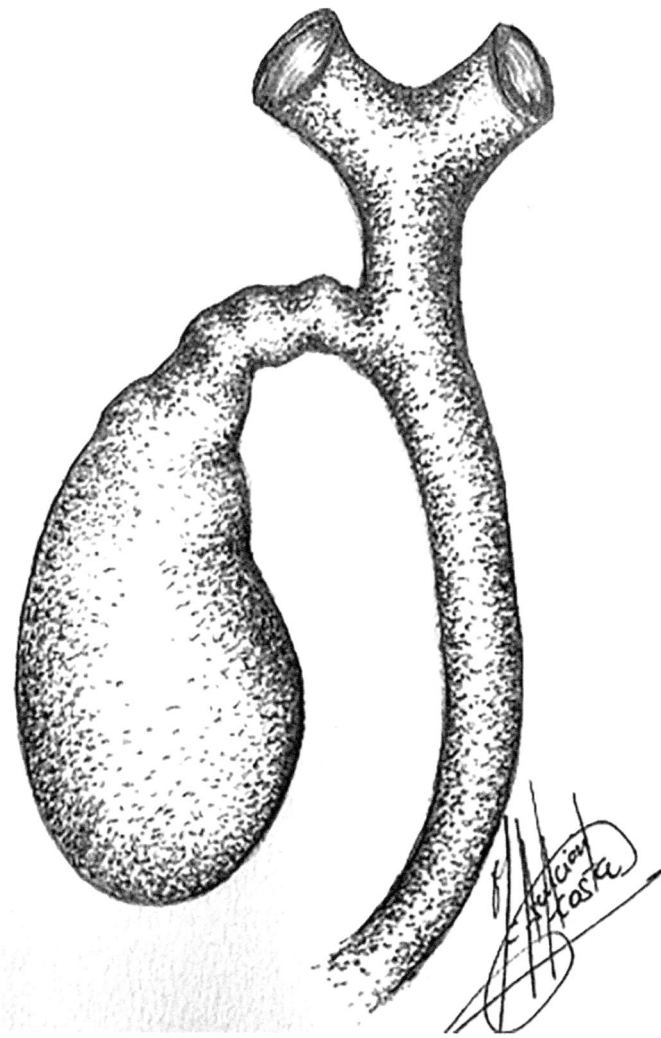

FIGURE 6.17 Both the cystic duct and CBD are dilated

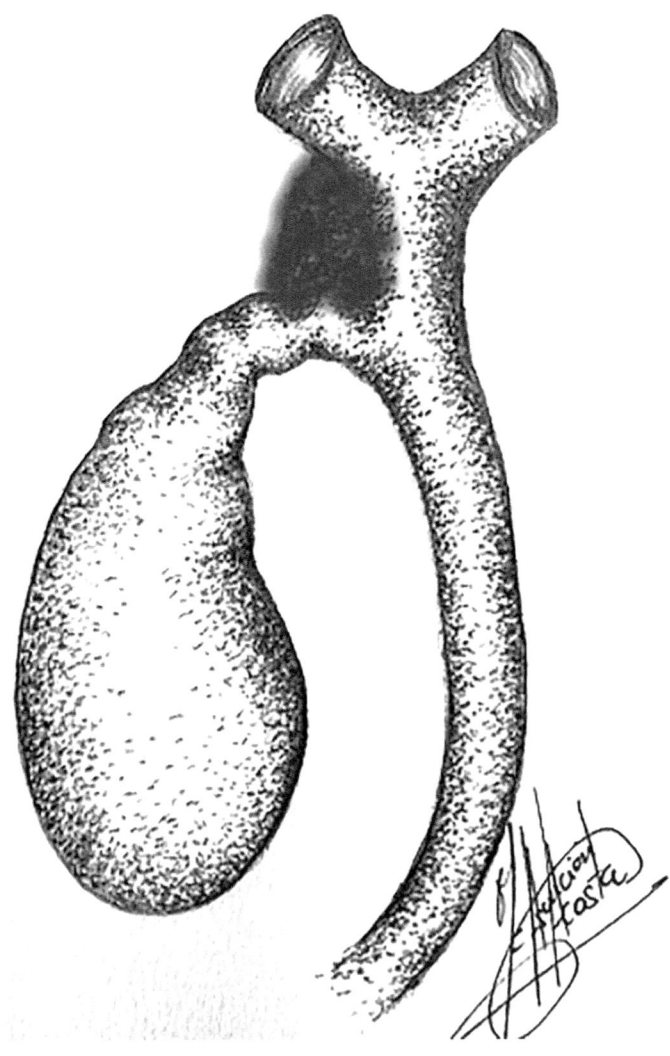

FIGURE 6.18 The frozen hilum

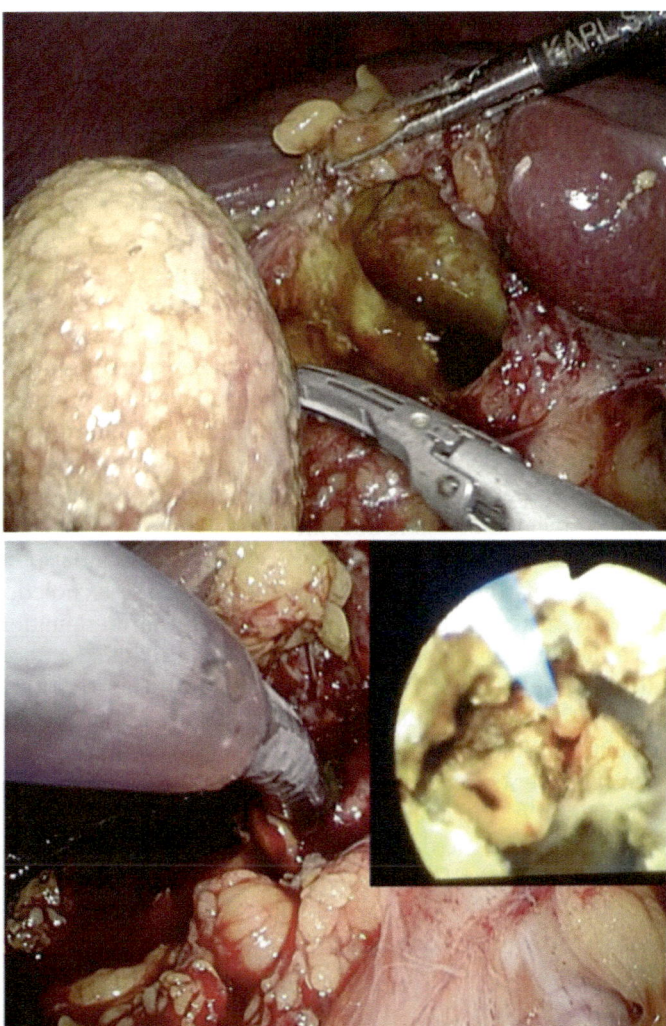

FIGURE 6.19 The impossible hilum requiring a transinfundibular approach (TIA) to the CBD combined with laser lithotripsy

At the time of describing the technique, we reviewed the last 154 consecutive patients in our series (February 2014–June 2018) and reported nine cases where the bile duct had been accessed through this novel route. For access, a cholecystotomy is performed at the infundibulum where generally a large stone or stones is/are impacted. Once the impacted stones are removed, the choledochoscope is then inserted with the tip directed to the infundibulum, and it often follows into the duct (Fig. 6.20). In our series of patients who underwent TIA, a cholangiogram was performed in only four patients, confirming that a cholangiogram is not necessary to perform this technique. However, we have used this technique more recently to achieve a cholangiogram in complex cases which would not be possible using the standard technique. A cholangiogram can be achieved either by injecting the contrast through the working channel of the choledochoscope or by guiding cystic duct intubation with the cholangiogram catheter during choledochoscopy. The TIA can also be used to clarify the anatomy and appropriately site a choledochotomy (if required). In a difficult hilum, transillumination from the tip of the scope can be used to identify the common bile duct, which in turn can be used to select the correct location for choledochotomy if this is required. In another patient, transillumination via the TIA (Fig. 6.21) was used to identify the entrance of the cystic duct into the CBD, allowing clarification of the anatomy and permitting further safe dissection of the cystic duct to subsequently perform our standard transcystic LBDE.

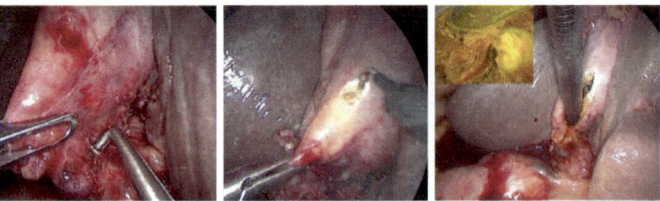

FIGURE 6.20 Technique for trans-infundibular approach (TIA) to the CBD. The impossible hilum (left), cholecystotomy (centre), TIA to the bile duct (right) with choledochoscopy (insert)

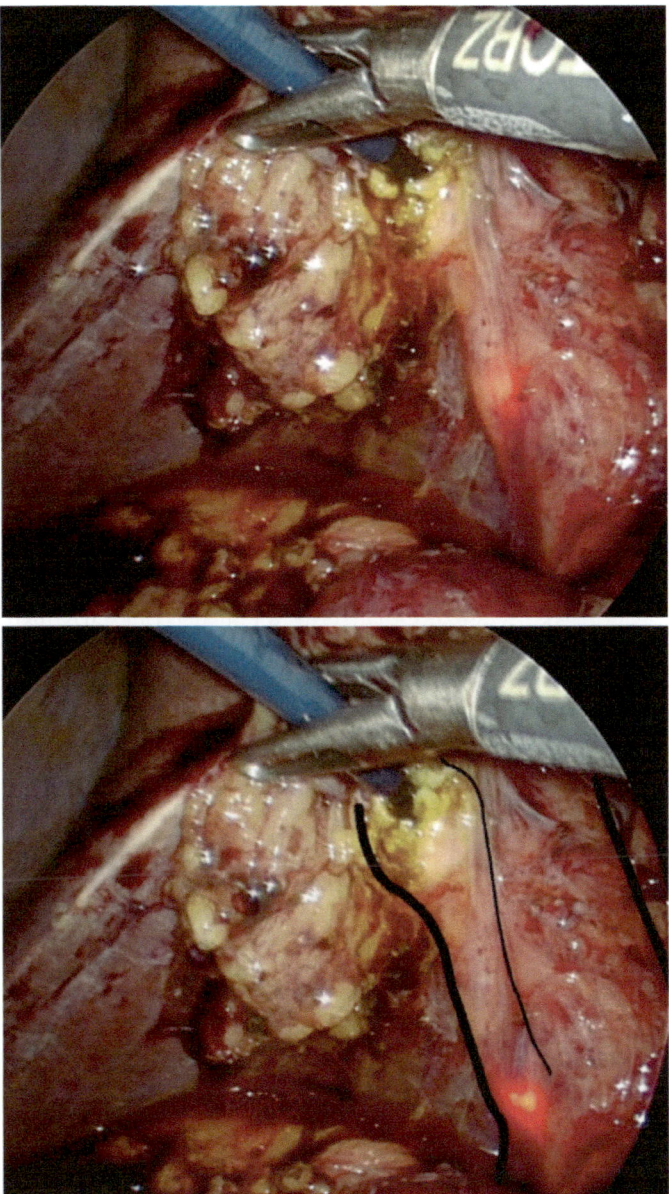

FIGURE 6.21 TIA used to clarify anatomy and delineate the cystic and common bile ducts

The management of complex cases, including type II Mirizzi syndrome, can be achieved laparoscopically using a combination of TIA and LABEL (TIA-LABEL). Type II Mirizzi syndrome (Fig. 6.22) is an uncommon cause of obstructive jaundice caused by an inflammatory response to

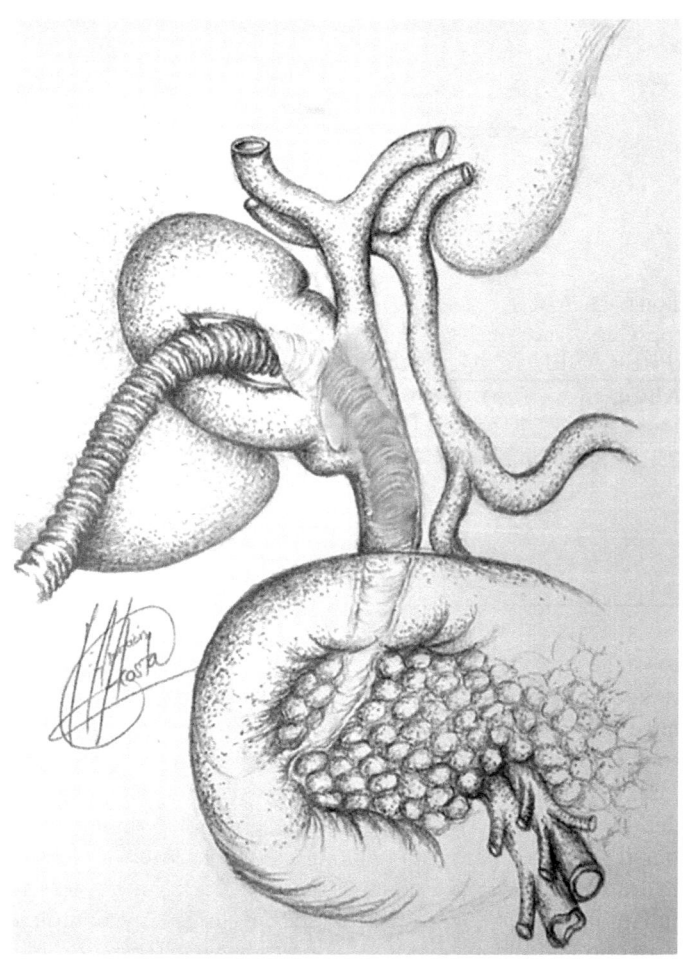

FIGURE 6.22 TIA in Type II Mirizzi syndrome

an impacted gallstone in Hartmann's pouch or the cystic duct with a resultant cholecystocholedochal fistula, which can sometimes be indistinguishable from a grossly dilated cystic duct. Figure 6.23 demonstrates complex type II Mirizzi syndrome in a patient that required a TIA-LABEL strategy. In this patient, a choledochotomy and bilioenteric anastomosis were considered but were ultimately not feasible options. The size of the stone (35 mm) and the high calcium content (as seen on pre-operative CT imaging) resulted in a prolonged laser lithotripsy time of over 6 h (total operative time 7.5 h). After comprehensive dusting and fragmentation of the stone with basket removal of the majority of fragments, some stone debris remained in the bile duct. After a lengthy procedure, we opted to clear the remaining fragments by a post-operative ERCP which was completed on the 14th post-operative day (the patient had normal LFTs post-operatively). In such cases, a pragmatic decision to complete CBD clearance with post-operative ERCP was appropriate as persisting with basket retrieval would have prolonged an already lengthy procedure.

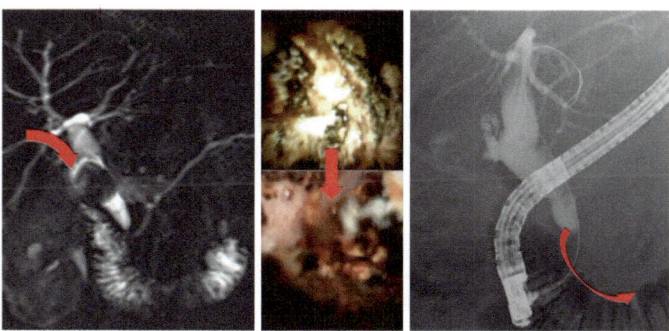

Figure 6.23 Trans-infundibular approach laser assisted bile duct exploration by laparoendoscopy (TIA-LABEL). Type II Mirizzi syndrome (left), lithotripsy of large stone (centre), post-operative ERCP to clear remaining fragments (right)

Closure After Accessing the Bile Duct

Closure of the Choledochotomy

Closure of choledochotomy can be performed in several ways:

1. Closure over a T-tube
2. Closure over an antegrade stent
3. Primary closure (without transcystic drain)
4. Primary closure with transcystic drain
5. Bilioenteric anastomosis

Closure Over a T-Tube

The T-tube should be trimmed in a similar way that is used in open surgery and it can be introduced into the abdominal cavity using the 10–12 mm port. After introducing the short arms into the bile duct proximally and distally (Fig. 6.24 left and centre), it is important to check that the drain moves freely within the duct. The main stem of the drain is exteriorised through the 5 mm right upper quadrant port (the same used for the choledochoscope). The choledochotomy is then closed over the T-tube with interrupted or running 5-0 Vicryl™ (Ethicon, New Brunswick, New Jersey, USA) on a round needle, starting either from the top or the bottom

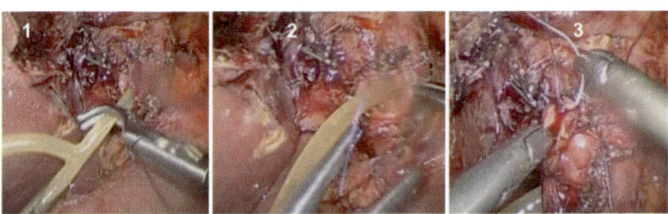

FIGURE 6.24 Closure of choledochotomy over a T-tube. Introduction proximally (left), distally (centre) and closure with interrupted sutures (right)

(Fig. 6.24 right). To test the closure, water can be injected into the T-tube at low pressure to ensure that there is no leak. The exteriorised main stem of the T-tube should be securely fixed to the skin with silk in multiple places to prevent inadvertent misplacement of the drain.

At the beginning of our LBDE series, closure of choledochotomy with T-tube was the favoured technique, however, its routine use was largely abandoned after the early years. Despite this, we still think there are some valid indications for its use: the presence of a choledochoduodenal or cholecystocholedochal fistula (including some instances of type 2 Mirizzi syndrome) and presence of certain types of choledochal cysts. Figure 6.25 illustrates the placement of a T-tube through a choledochotomy with the main stem exiting through a cholecystocholedochal fistula whilst the choledochotomy was closed independently. Figure 6.26 demonstrates reconstruction of the bile duct after resection of a type VI choledochal cyst (isolated dilation of the cystic duct). The technical considerations in this case consisted of resecting the saccular dilatation of the cystic duct (Fig. 6.26 right) and due to the wide implantation of the cystic duct, reconstruction of the bile duct over a T-tube with a subsequent ERCP-ES to address the common bilio-pancreatic channel associated in such cases. The insert (bottom right) in Fig. 6.26 is the choledochoscopic view showing the exit of the distal common bile duct into the common channel with entrance to the pancreatic duct (left) and duodenal papilla (right) [13].

Closure Over an Antegrade Stent

At the author's institution, routine use of T-tube for choledochotomy closure was abandoned in November 2001, and over the next decade or so, closure over an antegrade stent became the preferred choice of choledochotomy closure using a 7F Amsterdam stent. Antegrade insertion of the stent over a PTFE guidewire (0.035-inch diameter, 145 cm length, 3 cm flexible tip) (Cook Medical) (Chap. 4, Table 4.1, Serial

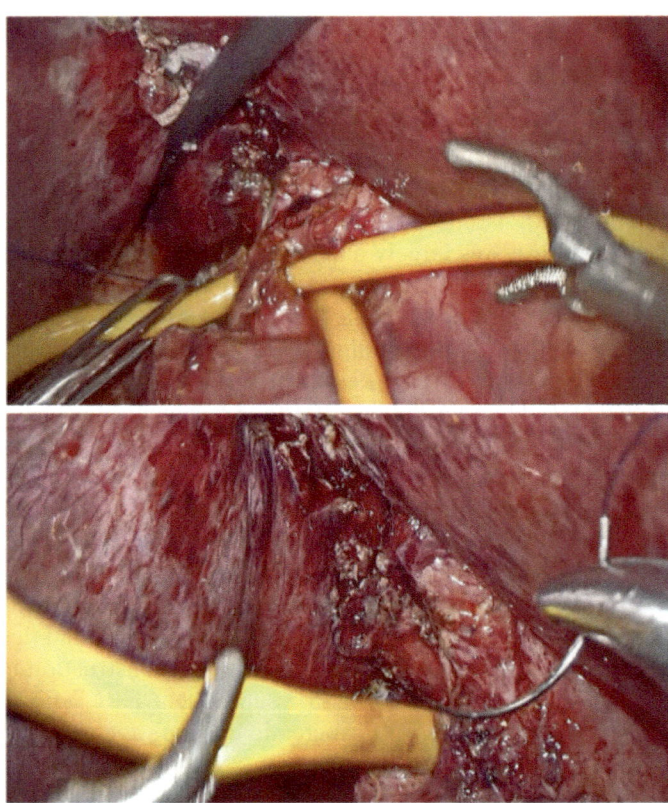

FIGURE 6.25 Use of a T-tube for a cholecystocholedochochal fistula

10) which was previously inserted into the CBD and duodenum under choledochoscopic view. The choledochoscope can also be railroaded over the guidewire after the stent thereby using the scope as a 'pusher' [14] and allowing direct visual confirmation that the stent has passed the papilla (Fig. 6.27). Following this, the choledochotomy can be closed over the stent with 5-0 Vicryl™. The stent is then removed after 2 or 3 weeks with an standard gastroscope and a snare (Fig. 6.28).

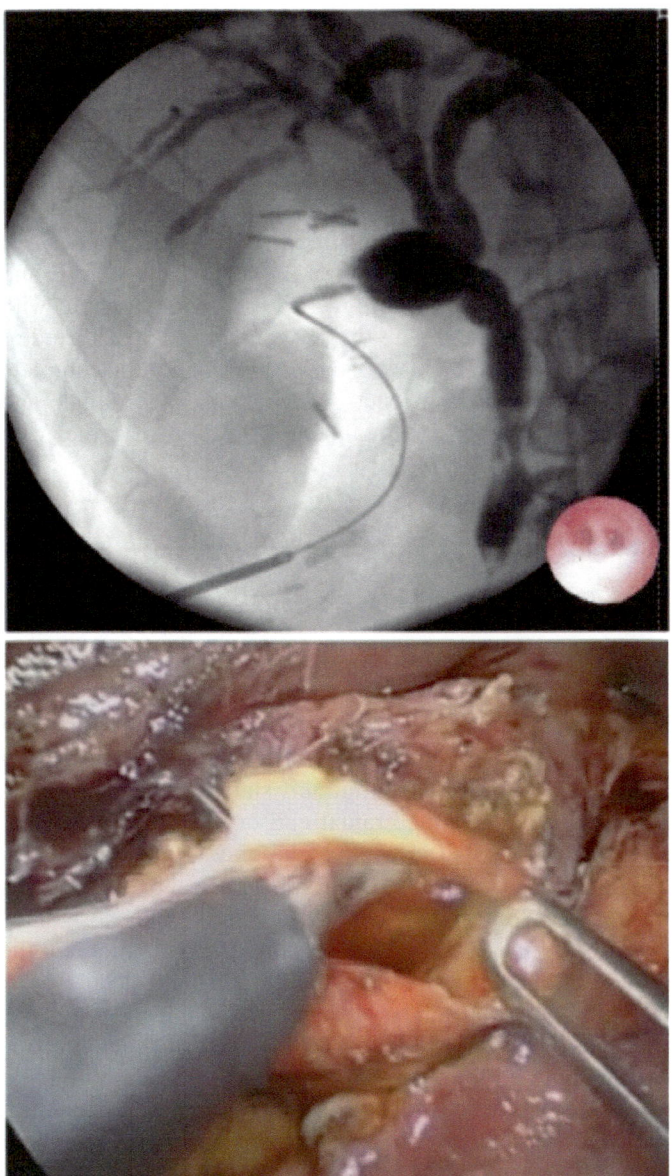

FIGURE 6.26 Type VI choledochal cyst

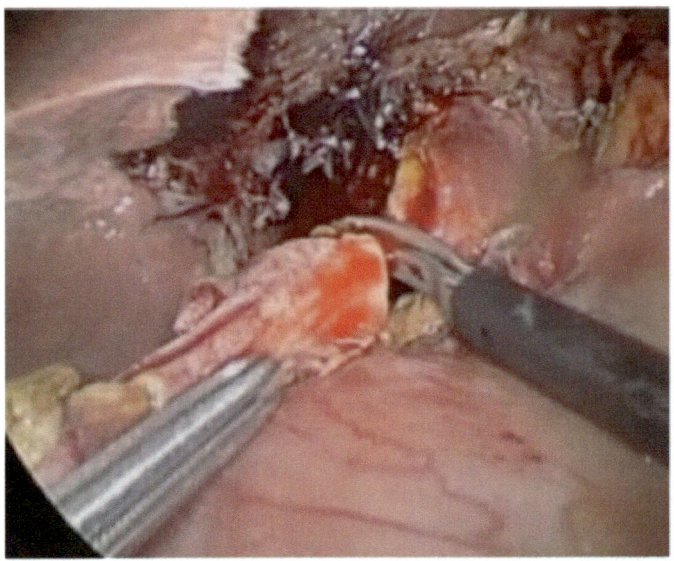

Figure 6.26 (continued)

Primary Closure (Without Transcystic Drain)

Since 2012, primary closure has been our preferred method of closure after choledochotomy. Our technique is performed using 5-0 Vicryl™ and we routinely start the closure by placing a stay suture at the cranial end of the choledochotomy (Fig. 6.29) [15, 16]. The choledochotomy is then closed primarily using a continuous suture on a curved needle starting from the caudal end, which is then tied to the originally placed stay suture (Fig. 6.30). It is important to maintain the tension after each stitch to ensure a water-tight closure.

Even though primary closure after choledochotomy is considered the preferred method of closure, it should only be used without additional biliary drainage when it is safe to do so. This can be checked by performing a completion intra-operative cholangiogram or cholangioscopy. Favourable

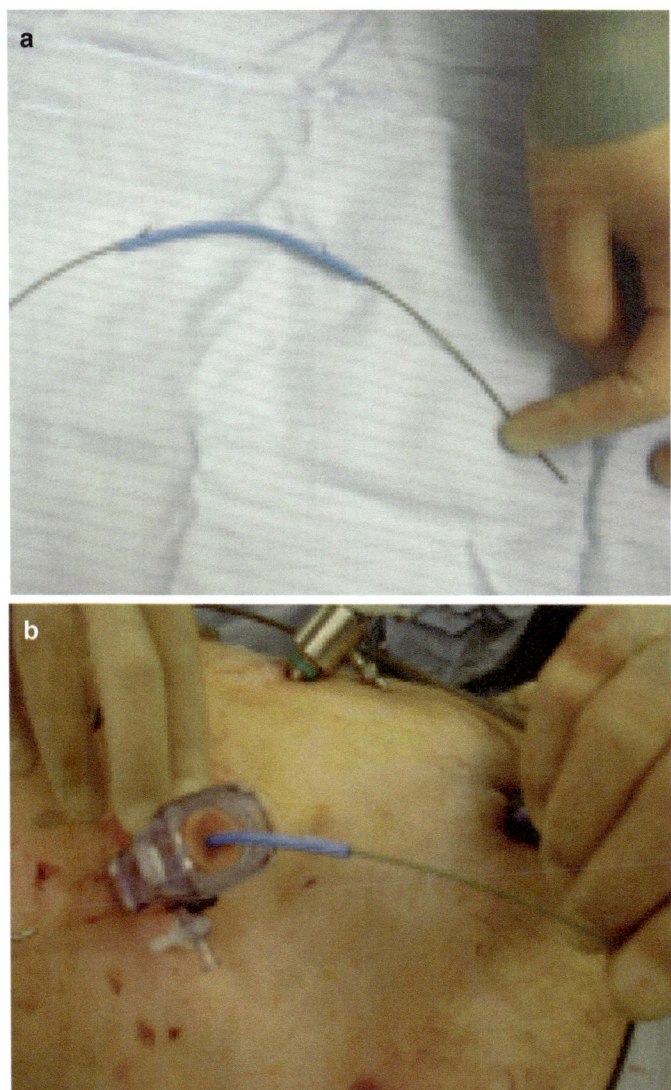

FIGURE 6.27 Insertion of antegrade stent

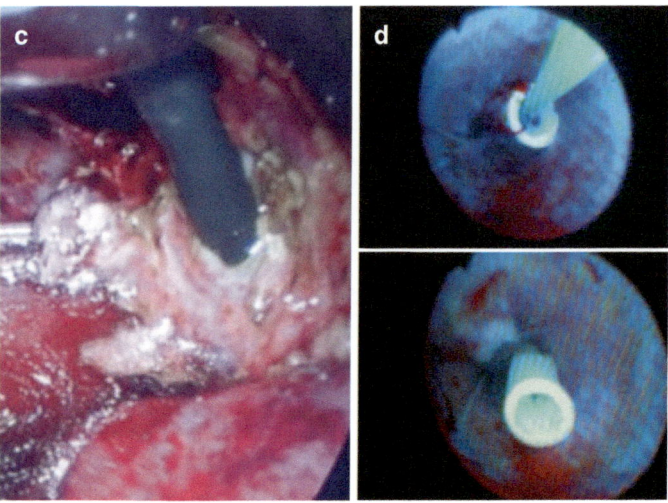

FIGURE 6.27 (continued)

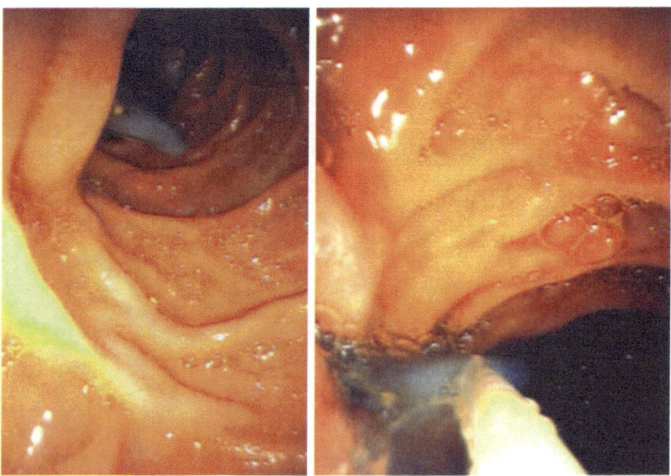

FIGURE 6.28 Removal of stent with gastroscope

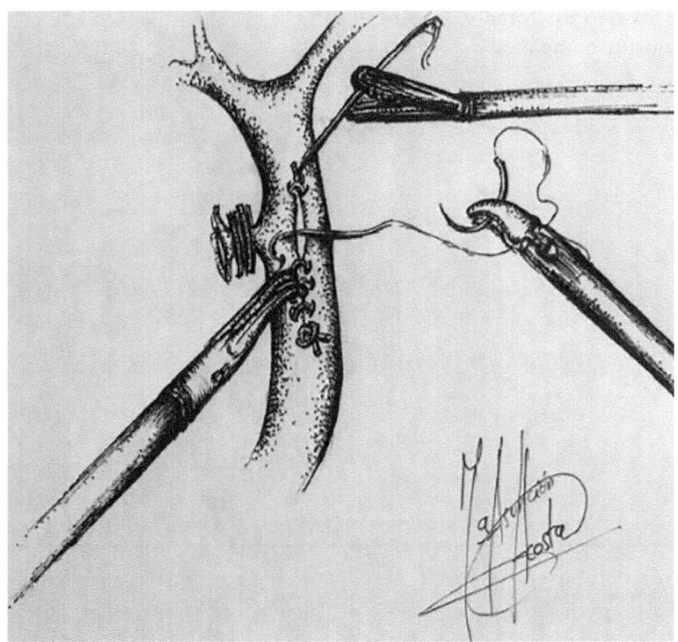

FIGURE 6.29 Start of the primary closure

observations to be able to proceed with primary closure (without transcystic drain) are that the duct is clear and that there is good passage into the duodenum. This can be seen under direct vision, passing the closed basket into the duodenum and then pulling the opened basket back, whilst watching to see how easily the papilla opens (Fig. 6.31). When we use the 3 mm choledochoscope, we often pass it directly into the duodenum (Fig. 6.32). If drainage into the duodenum is not satisfactory, it would be wise to use some form of bile duct decompression before closing the choledochotomy primarily. For this we favour an 8F drain placed transcystically (transcystic drain).

FIGURE 6.30 Primary closure completed

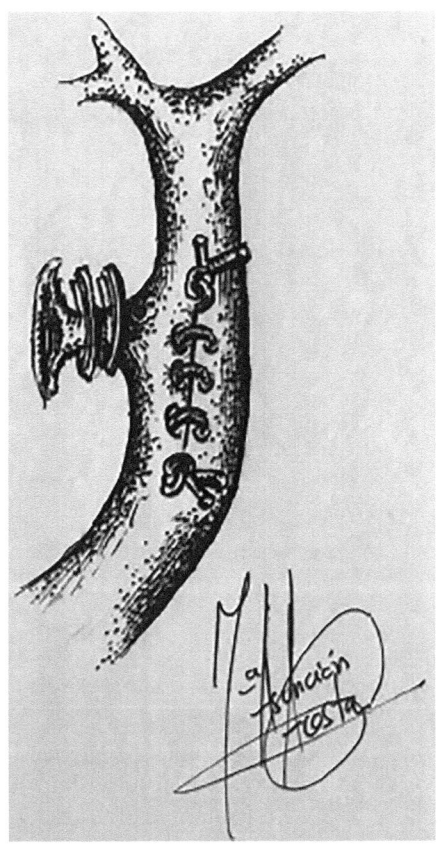

Primary Closure with Trancystic Drain

Primary closure with transcystic drain is a useful technique when it is highly desirable to protect the ductal closure in high-risk patients where the burden of a bile leak would have serious impact on morbidity and even mortality. It is also used when impaired papillary drainage is suspected rendering the bile duct a high-pressure system until normal outflow is once again established (Fig. 6.33). An 8F infant feeding tube or similar can be used for this and the tube is placed

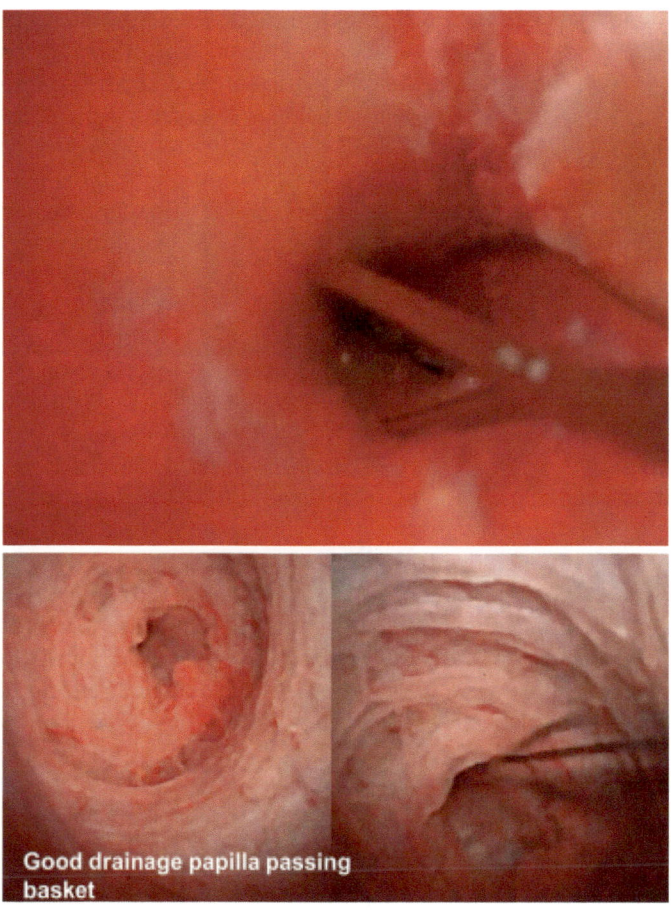

Good drainage papilla passing basket

FIGURE 6.31 Assessing the drainage of the bile duct under direct vision by choledochoscopy

transcystically, often railroaded over a guidewire (once the tip has been cut), so that the tip lies within the common bile duct. The drain should be secured well to the cystic duct stump using a 2-0 Vicryl™ intracorporeal tie. As with the T-tube, the extracorporeal part of the drain needs to be secured well to the skin in multiple places to avoid the drain becoming dis-

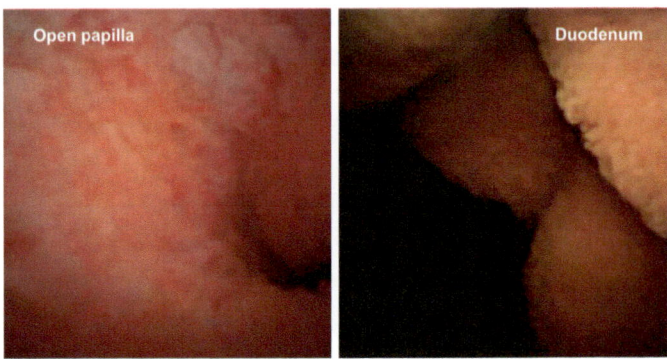

FIGURE 6.32 Passing the 3 mm choledochoscope through the papilla into the duodenum

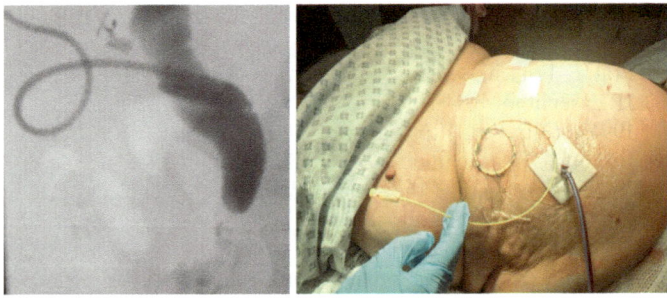

FIGURE 6.33 Primary closure with transcystic drain in a patient with papillary oedema

lodged. The transcystic drain is better tolerated than the T-tube and is also subject to less complications.

Bilioenteric Anastomosis

Rarely after the choledochotomy and bile duct exploration we need to perform a choledochoduodenostomy. The indications include retained, recurrent and impacted bile duct stones, strictures of the bile duct, stenosis of the sphincter of Oddi, pancreatitis associated with biliary disease, choledochal cysts, fistulas of the bile duct and biliary obstruction, either benign or malignant. The laparoscopic technique is similar to that performed in open surgery. A vertical incision is made in the supraduodenal portion of the common bile duct and a similar-sized transverse incision in the duodenum. Two stay sutures are placed, one lateral and one medial, bringing the two openings together (Fig. 6.34 left). The stay sutures are then placed under traction and exteriorised using an Endo Close™ (Fig. 6.34 left). The posterior layer of the anastomosis is performed first (Fig. 6.34 right), historically using interrupted 4-0 Vicryl™ but a contemporary alternative would be to use a continuous V-Loc™ suture (Covidien, Mansfield, Massachusetts, USA). Once the posterior layer is completed, the stay sutures can then be tied and then the anterior layer of the anastomosis completed in a similar fashion to the posterior layer (Fig. 6.35).

Closure After the Transcystic Approach

Closure after transcystic exploration is often indistinguishable from that after a laparoscopic cholecystectomy without bile duct exploration. An Endoloop (Ethicon, New Brunswick, New Jersey, USA) or sometimes just a clip is needed to close the cystic duct stump (Fig. 6.36). If a completion cholangiogram is indicated and the cholangiogram catheter is placed once again transcystically, a loose 2-0 Vicryl™ tie can be placed around the cystic duct to prevent leakage of contrast, which can then be tightened once the catheter is removed to achieve secure closure of the cystic duct (Fig. 6.37).

At the junction between the cystic and common bile duct there is often a saccular dilatation. If the cystic duct cannot be cannulated for the standard transcystic approach, then this dilatation may have to be used for access to the bile duct. This can complicate the closure and often requires sutures. The same will occur if a near-total cholecystectomy is performed after the TIA approach (Fig. 6.38). In this scenario, the infundibulum should be closed under direct vision of the entrance

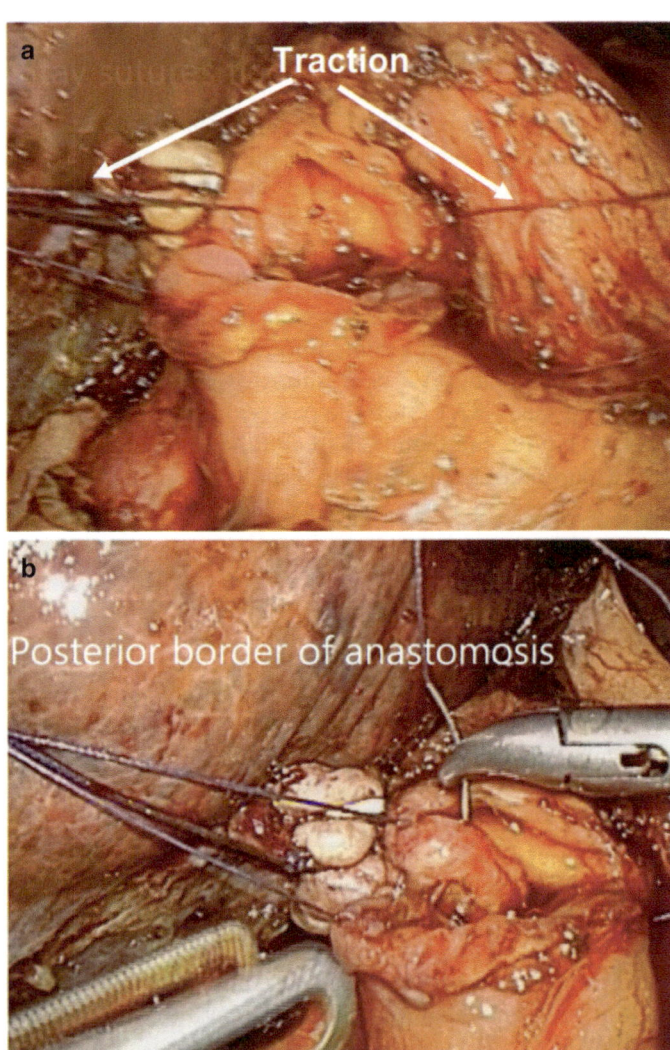

FIGURE 6.34 Choledochoduodenostomy. (**a**) placement of stay sutures for traction and to bring the two openings together. (**b**) performing the posterior layer of the anastomosis

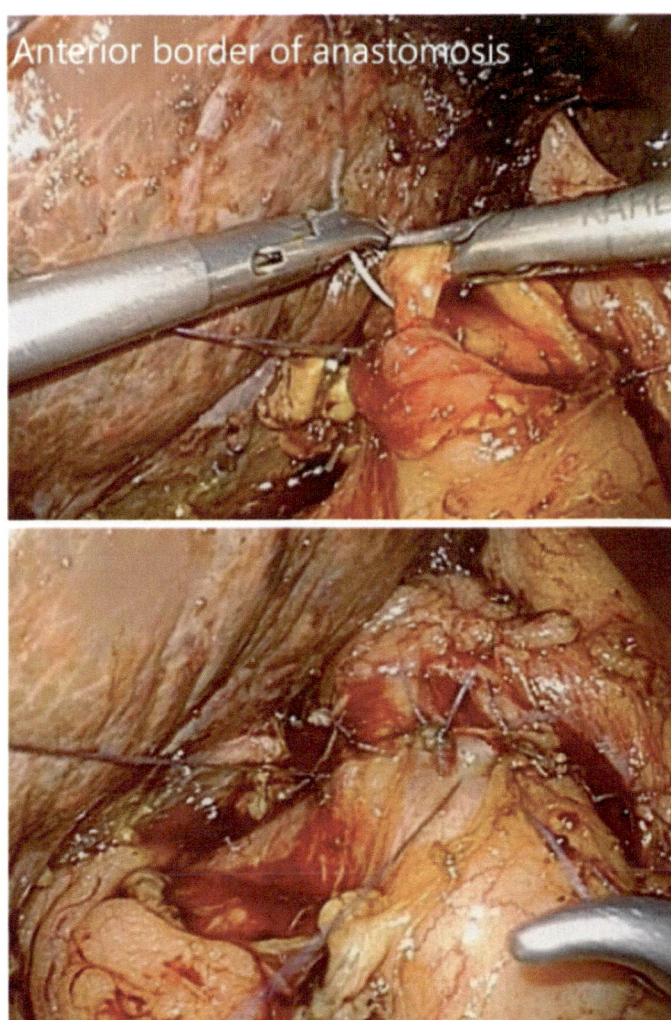

FIGURE 6.35 Choledochoduodenostomy: anterior layer

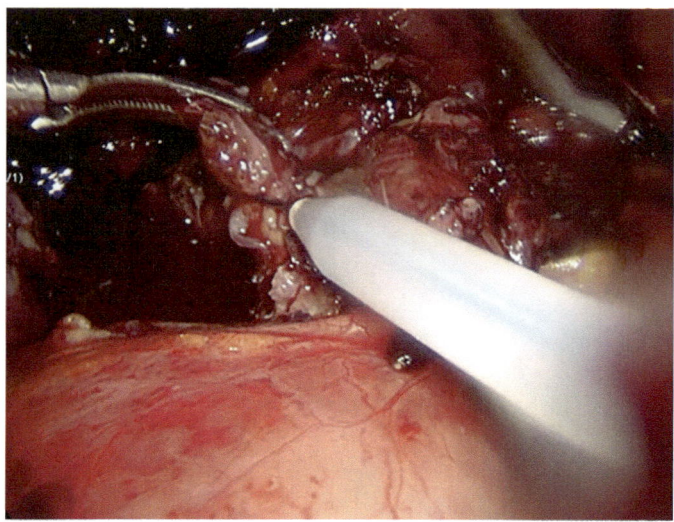

FIGURE 6.36 Closure of the cystic duct stump with an Endoloop

of the cystic duct (Fig. 6.38 blue arrow) or with the 3 mm disposable choledochoscope inside of the bile duct to avoid stenosis.

Bile Duct Exploration in the Patient with Roux-En-Y Gastric Bypass (RYGB)

Approximately 10–30% of patients develop cholelithiasis (of which about a third are symptomatic) and >1% develop choledocholithiasis after bariatric surgery [17–20]. Following laparoscopic Roux-en-Y gastric bypass (LRYGB) specifically, the incidence is slightly higher. Although it is not our practice, the majority of patients with choledocholithiasis and concomitant gallstones in the UK still receive pre-operative ERCP. Because of surgically altered anatomy, traditional trans-oral ERCP is not possible in patients with RYGB. Various techniques have been described to access the biliary tree in patients with altered anatomy or in situations where tradi-

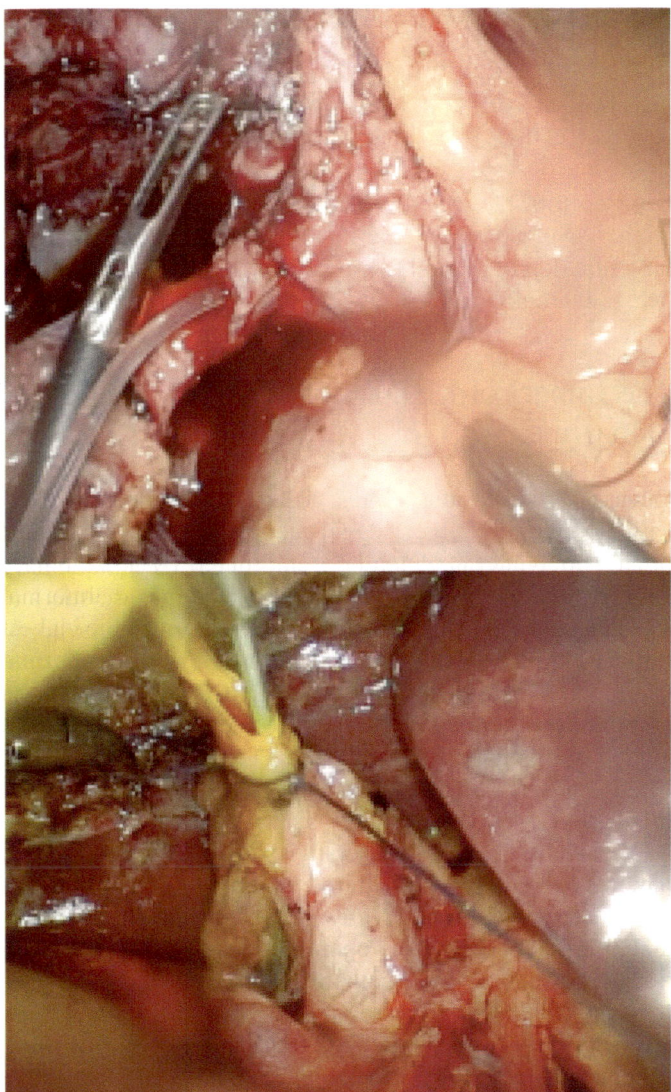

FIGURE 6.37 Completion intra-operative cholangiogram prior to cystic duct closure using an intracorporeal 2-0 Vicryl™ tie

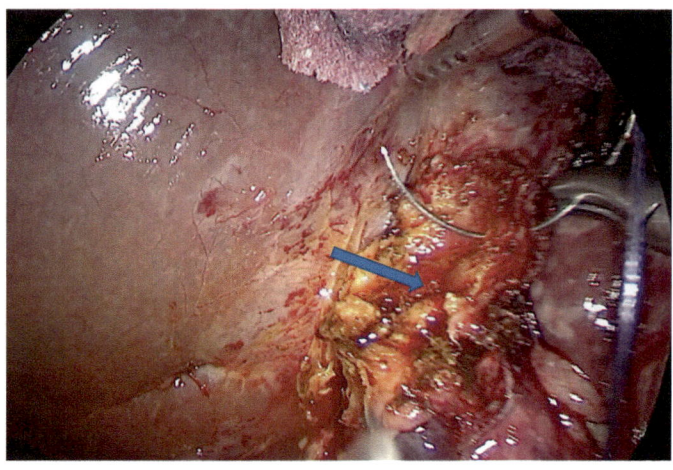

FIGURE 6.38 Closure after TIA

tional ERCP has failed. Varied results of each technique have been reported. The various options include transcystic and transductal LBDE, laparoscopic choledochoduodenostomy, Laparoscopic   Transgastric   Endoscopic   Retrograde Cholangiopancreatography (LTG-ERCP), single-balloon enteroscopy-assisted ERCP, endoscopic ultrasound (EUS) guided transhepatic ERCP, EUS guided rendezvous and percutaneous transhepatic cholangiography (with or without lithotripsy).

The technique for transcystic or transductal LBDE in patients with surgically altered anatomy in the same as described above. Post-operative adhesions are usually minimal after LRYGB, but the operating surgeon should be cautious upon induction of pneumoperitoneum in these patients. It is our opinion that transcystic LBDE is the optimal management strategy for all patients with choledocholithiasis and concomitant gallstones, including patients with surgically altered anatomy. LTG-ERCP has a post-operative complication rate of 36% [21] compared with lower complication rates of up to 17% for other techniques [16, 22–24] (Table 6.2). Accompanying a very high post-procedure complication rate for LTG-ERCP is a 6% rate of conversion to open surgery

TABLE 6.2 Various techniques to access the biliary tree in patients with altered anatomy and their respective major post-operative complication rate

Technique	Major post-operative complications (%)
Transcystic LBDE	1
Transductal LBDE	7
Laparoscopic choledochoduodenostomy	9
LTG-ERCP	13
Single-balloon enteroscopy-assisted ERCP	7
Percutaneous transhepatic removal	7

LBDE laparoscopic bile duct exploration; *LTG-ERCP* Laparoscopic Transgastric Endoscopic Retrograde Cholangiopancreatography, *ERCP* endoscopic retrograde cholangiopancreatography

and 10% requiring a further surgical procedure. Regarding single-balloon enteroscopy-assisted ERCP, biliary cannulation and procedural success rates are 90% and 76% respectively [23]. Our own institutional data reports success rates of 99% for transcystic LBDE in all patients and 100% for patients with surgically altered anatomy.

References

1. Qandeel H, Zino S, Hanif Z, Nassar MKNA. Basket-in-catheter access for transcystic laparoscopic bile duct exploration: technique and results. Surg Endosc. 2016;30:1958–64.
2. Xiao-Bin Y, An-Shu X, Jian-Gang L, Yong-Ping X, De-Song X, Chao-Chun F, et al. Dilation of the cystic duct confluence in laparoscopic common bile duct exploration and stone extraction in patients with secondary choledocholithiasis. BMC Surg. 2020; Mar 17:20.
3. Mortelé KJ, Ros PR. Anatomic variants of the biliary tree: MR cholangiographic findings and clinical applications. Am J Roentgenol. 2001;177:389–99.

4. Dion YM, Rattele R, Morin J, Gravel D. Common bile duct exploration: the place of laparoscopic choledochotomy. Surg Laparosc Endosc. 1994;4:419–24.

5. Gigot JF, Navez B, Etienne J, Cambier E, Jadoul GP, et al. A stratified intraoperative surgical strategy is mandatory during laparoscopic common bile duct exploration for common bile duct stones. Lessons and limits from an initial experience of 92 patients. Surg Endosc. 1997;11:722–8.

6. Martin IJ, Bailey IS, Rhodes M, O'Rourke N, Nathanson L, Fielding G. Towards T-tube free laparoscopic bile duct exploration: a methodologic evolution during 300 consecutive procedures. Ann Surg. 1998;228:29–34.

7. Navarro-Sánchez A, Ashrafian H, Segura-Sampedro J, Martrinez-Isla A. LABEL procedure: laser-assisted bile duct exploration by Laparoendoscopy for choledocholithiasis: improving surgical outcomes and reducing technical failure. Surg Endosc. 2017;31(5):2103–8.

8. Jones T, Al Musawi J, Navaratne L, Martinez-Isla A. Holmium laser lithotripsy improves the rate of successful transcystic laparoscopic common bile duct exploration. Langenbeck's Arch Surg. 2019;404(8):985–92.

9. Martínez Cecilia D, Valenti-Azcárate V, Qurashi K, Garcia-Agustí A, Marrtinez-isla A. Ventajas de la coledocorrafia laparoscópica sobre el stent. Experiencia tras seis años. Cir Esp. 2008;84(2):78–82.

10. Martinez-Isla A, Martinez Cecilia D, Vilaça J, Navaratne L, Navarro Sanchez A. Laser-assisted bile duct exploration using laparoendoscopy LABEL technique, different scenarios and technical details. Epublication Websurgcom [Internet]. 2018;18(03) Available from: http://websurg.com/doi/vd01en5197

11. Navaratne L, Al-Musawi J, Acosta-Mérida A, Vilaça J, Martinez-Isla A. Trans-infundibular choledochoscopy: a method for accessing the common bile duct in complex cases. Langenbeck's Arch Surg. 2018;403(6):777–83.

12. Williams E, Beckingham I, El Sayed G, et al. Updated guideline on the management of common bile duct stones (CBDS). Gut. 2017;66:765–82.

13. Navarro-Sánchez A, Ashrafian H, Martínez-Isla A. An abnormal intraoperative cholangiogram. JAMA Surg. 2015;150(10):1009.

14. Isla A, Griniatsos J, Wan A. A technique for safe placement of a biliary endoprosthesis after laparoscopic choledochotomy. J Laparoendosc Adv Surg Tech [Internet]. 2002;12(3):207–11. Available from: http://www.liebertpub.com/doi/10.1089/10926420260188128

15. Abellán Morcillo I, Qurashi K, Isla ACJAM. Tubo de Kehr Stent Cierre primario L. Exploración laparoscópica de la vía biliar, lecciones aprendidas tras más de 200 casos. Cir Esp [Internet]. 2014;9(5):3–4. Available from: www.elsevier.es/cirugia%5Cnhttp://dx.doi.org/10.1016/j.ciresp.2013.02.010%5Cnhttp://www.elsevier.es

16. Navaratne L, Martinez-Isla A. Transductal versus transcystic laparoscopic common bile duct exploration: an institutional review of over four hundred cases. Surg Endosc. 2021;35(1):437–48. https://doi.org/10.1007/s00464-020-07522.

17. Tapas M, Kona Kumari L, Kiran KP. Prevalence of cholelithiasis and choledocholithiasis in morbidly obese south Indian patients and the further development of biliary calculus disease after sleeve gastrectomy, gastric bypass and mini gastric bypass. Obes Surg. 2016;26(10):2411–7.

18. Nagem R, Lazaro-da-Silva A, Morroni de Oliveira R, Garcia Morato V. Gallstone-related complications after Roux-en-Y gastric bypass: a prospective study. Hepatobiliary Pancreat Dis Int 2012;15(11(6)):630–5.

19. Tucker ON, Fajwaks P, Szomstein S, Rosenthal R. Is concomitant cholecystectomy necessary in obese patients undergoing laparoscopic gastric bypass surgery? Surg Endosc. 2008;22(11):2450–4.

20. Warschkow R, Tarantino I, Ukegjini K, Beutner U, Guller U, Schmied B, et al. Concomitant cholecystectomy during laparoscopic roux-en-Y gastric bypass in obese patients is not justified: a meta-analysis. Obes Surg. 2013;23(3):397–407.

21. Frederiksen N, Tveskov L, Helgstrand F, Naver L, Floyd A. Treatment of common bile duct stones in gastric bypass patients with laparoscopic transgastric endoscopic retrograde cholangiopancreatography. Obes Surg. 2017;27(6):1409–13.

22. DuCoin C, Moon R, Teixeira A, Jawad M. Laparoscopic choledochoduodenostomy as an alternate treatment for common bile duct stones after Roux-en-Y gastric bypass. Surg Obes Relat Dis. 2014;10(4):652–3.

23. Tanisaka Y, Ryozawa S, Mizuide M, Araki R, Fujita A, Ogawa T, et al. Status of single-balloon enteroscopy-assisted endoscopic retrograde cholangiopancreatography in patients with surgically altered anatomy: Systematic review and meta-analysis on biliary interventions. dig endosc. 2020;online ahe.

24. Ozcan N, Kahriman G, Mavili E. Percutaneous transhepatic removal of bile duct stones: results of 261 patients. Cardiovasc Interv Radiol. 2012;35(3):621–7.

Chapter 7
Our Experience of Laparoscopic Bile Duct Exploration from Nearly 500 Cases: Leveraging Access to Technology and Enhanced Surgical Technique (LATEST) and the Biliary Surgery 2.0 Concept

Alberto Martinez-Isla, Lalin Navaratne, and María Asunción Acosta-Mérida

A. Martinez-Isla (✉) · L. Navaratne
Northwick Park and St Mark's Hospitals, London North West
University Healthcare NHS Trust, London, UK
e-mail: a.isla@imperial.ac.uk; lalin.navaratne@doctors.org.uk

M. A. Acosta-Mérida
General Surgery Department, Hospital Universitario de Gran
Canaria Doctor Negrín,
Las Palmas de Gran Canaria, Las Palmas, Spain

© The Author(s), under exclusive license to Springer Nature   201
Switzerland AG 2022
A. Martinez-Isla, L. Navaratne (eds.), *Laparoscopic Common
Bile Duct Exploration*, In Clinical Practice,
https://doi.org/10.1007/978-3-030-93203-9_7

Our Series

As discussed in Chap. 2, Laparoscopic Bile Duct Exploration (LBDE) is considered a valid option, if not the option of choice, in the management of ductal stones with gallbladder in situ. Outcomes used to compare it with the other treatment modalities include clearance rate, retained stones, morbidity and hospital stay (Table 7.1). As expected, mortality is very low in all approaches, and therefore is often not used as a parameter to compare different treatment options [1].

Approximately two-fifths (44%) of the patients within our series presented with jaundice and almost one-fifth (17%) with acute pancreatitis [2]. This is comparable to previously published large series of LBDE. Zhu et al., published their cohort of 708 patients and reported similar presentations with 39% and 20% respectively [3]. Table 7.1 summarises the main outcomes (CBD clearance, morbidity, mortality and hospital stay) following two-stage (pre-operative ERCP followed by laparoscopic cholecystectomy) and one-stage (laparoscopic cholecystectomy with LBDE) management of choledocholithiasis with concomitant gallstones from the literature (systematic reviews and randomised trials) and compares these metrics with data from our own series of LBDE [4–10].

CBD Clearance

The CBD clearance rate of 96.4% that has been achieved in our series compares favourably with the published standard. Moreover, treatment success was 100% from the last 100 patients (Table 7.1). The last failure of stone extraction within our series was case number 287 out of 481. Furthermore, a fifth of the patients in our series had previously undergone failed endoscopic retrograde cholangiopancreatography (ERCP). We have analysed potential causes of stone extraction failure during LBDE and found that it was mainly due to distal impacted stones [11]. In addition to the outcomes listed

TABLE 7.1 Outcomes of pre-operative ERCP + LC (ERCP-LC) and LCBDE at the time of LC (LC + LCBDE) from the literature, our series of over 400 patients and the last 100 patients from our series

Outcome	Study	ERCP-LC	LC + LCBDE	Our series	Our series last 100 patients
CBD clearance	Liu[a]	89.1%	92.7% (p = 0.03)	96.8%	100% (90% transcystic)
	Zhu[a]	85.7%	90.2% (p = 0.03)		
	Singh[a]	82.2%	88.1% (p = 0.02)		
	Prasson[a]	78.8%	82% (p = 0.15)		
	Noble[b]	61.7%	100% (p < 0.001)		
Morbidity	Liu[a]	18.8%	15.4% (p = 0.58)	18.7% (8% transcystic)	10%
	Zhu[a]	14.2%	15.3% (p = 0.52)		
	Singh[a]	14.6%	13.9% (p = 0.84)		
Bile leak	Liu[a]	0.5%	6.3%	3.8% (0.57% transcystic)	1%
	Zhu[a]	1.3%	8.1% (p = 0.0005)		
Pancreatitis	Liu[a]	3.6%	0.3%	3.8% (1% transcystic)	0%
	Zhu[a]	3.5%	0.5% (p = 0.008)		

(continued)

TABLE 7.1 (continued)

Outcome	Study	ERCP-LC	LC + LCBDE	Our series	Our series last 100 patients
Hospital stay	Liu[a]	–	WMD −3.32 days (p < 0.05)	2 days	1 day
	Zhu[a]	–	WMD −1.02 days (p = 0.04)		
	Singh[a]	6.5 ± 3.4 days	4.9 ± 1.6 days (p = 0.05)		
	Nagaraja[a]	5.85 days	4.65 days (p = 0.39)		
Mortality	Dasari[a]	1%	0.7% (p = 0.72)	0.6%	0%

WMD weighted mean difference
[a]Systematic review of randomised controlled trials
[b]Randomised controlled trial

in Table 7.1, we also need to consider the number of patients with stones inadvertently left behind (retained stones). In our series, we have found 4 out of 481 (~0.8%) patients with retained stones (August 2021) [2]. By comparison, this is less than that described in other series of LBDE, which have reported closer to 6% [10]. CBD stone recurrence is often difficult to evaluate accurately, because many of the patients feel well after the procedure and in most circumstances are not followed up beyond a couple of years. However, we were still able to identify a minority of patients (1.25%) with recurrent stones that is certainly less than the 14.1% reported in other series [12].

Since we started performing the technique in 1998, our main concern has always been failing to clear the bile duct of stones, and in our experience, the two main reasons behind this have been: (i) the presence of distal impacted stones and (ii) the existence of a proximal stenosis (precluding access to the stone with the choledochoscope +/− lithotripsy). In 2006, we published the reasons for failure of the laparoscopic technique, with a series of 60 patients at the time [11]. We defined failure as 'the impossibility of stone extraction from the lumen of the CBD' and defined an impacted stone as one which 'did not allow the passage of the Dormia basket across it' and 'could not be moved proximally or distally.' At that time, our success rate was 90%, far from the 100% obtained in the last ~200 cases. Of the six cases where CBD clearance was not achieved, one was converted to open surgery and the stone removed through a transduodenal approach; another required a mini-laparotomy for a hand-assisted disimpaction with further closure of the CBD over a T-tube; and four patients required post-operative ERCP, two of which had an antegrade stent passed beyond the stone into the duodenum during laparoscopy (Fig. 7.1). At that time, the transductal approach was our preferred approach [13, 14], far from what is widely recommended now [15, 16], and certainly not our own current opinion [2]. At the time, the recommended strategies to deal with impacted stones were: (i) balloon dilatation of the papilla [17], (ii) glucagon injection for relaxation of the

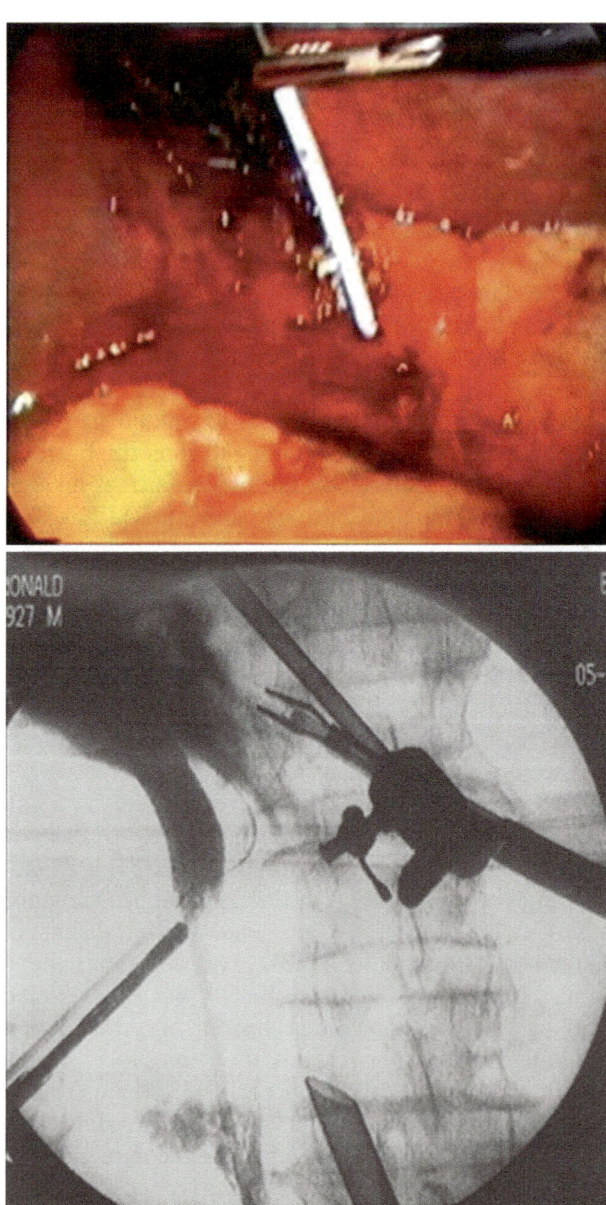

FIGURE 7.1 Insertion of an antegrade stent across an impacted stone

papilla [18], (iii) intra-operative or post-operative ERCP, (iv) antegrade sphincterotomy [19], (v) electrohydraulic lithotripsy (EHL) [20], or (vi) transoral laser lithotripsy [21]. The first option (i) is associated with a high rate of pancreatitis [22] and the use of lithotripsy was developed later at our institution. We found that the best way to treat impacted stones at the time was post-operative ERCP, either with intra-operative insertion of an antegrade stent across the stone (Fig. 7.1), or after closing the CBD over a T-tube or transcystic drain for decompression. Impacted stones continued to be a problem at our institution until February 2014 when we introduced the Lithotripsy-Assisted Bile duct Exploration by Laparoendoscopy (LABEL) technique [23, 24].

When we reported our outcomes from 416 patients since starting the technique in 1998, failure to clear the bile duct was analysed in four chronological groups of 104 patients. Clearance rate, as expected, improved after the first 100 cases, most likely due to the learning curve and equipment selection [2]. Conversion to open surgery due to LBDE failure soon disappeared and we learned to complete the procedure laparoscopically whilst able to alleviate any biliary obstruction [2]. However, there still remained a 2–3% failure rate, which would only be overcome in the last quartile of the series (Table 7.1). This was mainly due to the introduction of LABEL and being able to leverage other emerging technologies [2, 23, 25–27].

In our experience, the rate of inadvertently left (retained) stones was very low (<1%). In the last quartile of the current series (n = 120), where 92% transcystic LBDE rate was achieved, we did not experience difficulty in managing proximal bile duct (common hepatic duct) stones. We were able to achieve a proximal choledochoscopic view in over 70% of patients from the last quartile of the series. Furthermore, our threshold for performing choledochoscopy after an equivocal intra-operative cholangiogram has lowered as our transcystic rate has increased (Fig. 7.2). The blank (negative) choledochoscopy rate was 29% for the last quartile of the series as demonstrated in Fig. 7.2. This may be considered a high rate of negative choledochoscopy (with increased cost) but it is

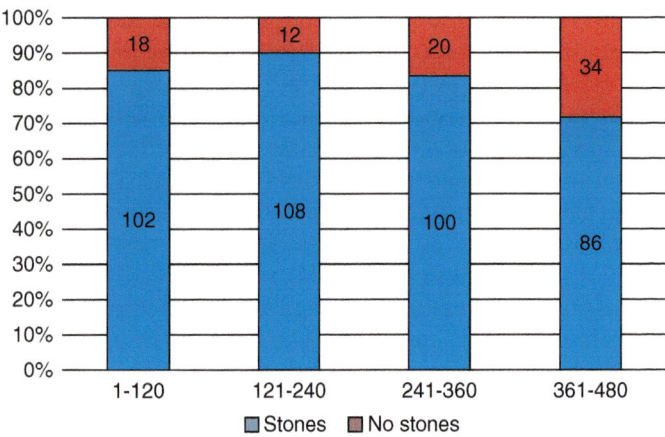

FIGURE 7.2 Rate of negative (blank) choledochoscopy with increased experience (480 cases)

certainly not at the expense of increased morbidity [13] due to the fact that most of those choledochoscopies were performed transcystically (97%) and completed with ultra-thin choledochoscopes (85%). Transcystic choledochoscopy with an ultra-thin choledochoscope does not result in additional morbidity compared to laparoscopic cholecystectomy alone. An even higher rate of negative choledochoscopy (41%) was experienced in the early days of this technique in 1985 by Brian Ashby, but at that time he was performing a choledochoscopy that not only required open surgery but also a choledochotomy to access the bile duct along with its associated morbidity [28].

Morbidity

Most studies to date, including systematic reviews of randomised trials, have failed to demonstrate difference in morbidity between LBDE at time of laparoscopic cholecystectomy and pre-operative ERCP followed by laparoscopic cholecystectomy [6, 7, 29–32]. In our experience, as summarised in

Table 7.1, morbidity is mainly represented by bile leak and pancreatitis, the latter mainly associated with the historical use of anterograde stents. Increased use of the transcystic approach has helped us to decrease the total morbidity from 21% (when the transductal route is used) to 8% (p = 0.0001) [2].

Bile leak is the most frequently occurring morbidity associated with LBDE, which in our series complicated 3.3% of patients (n = 481). As expected, bile leak was associated with closure of choledochotomy after the transductal approach. From 236 LBDE cases performed transcystically, bile leak occurred in only two patients (<1%). Furthermore, of the two bile leaks, one was secondary to a duct of Luschka and therefore related to the cholecystectomy part of the operation rather than the bile duct exploration [2]. These results are therefore acceptable when compared to the literature and certainly not a drawback for the technique [33].

The second most common complication associated with the technique is acute pancreatitis, with an incidence of 4% in our series (n = 481), which is mainly related to the closure of choledochotomy over an anterograde stent. This complication has been largely abolished since abandoning that practice and now we recommend using the transcystic approach where possible (avoiding choledochotomy altogether) or primary closure of choledochotomy when the transductal route is unavoidable [2]. This treatment strategy has also been shared by other authors [34, 35]. Our outcomes suggest that increased use of the transcystic approach coincides with reduced complications of LBDE, therefore strengthening the position of the single-stage management of choledocholithiasis against other treatment options (two-stage management: pre- or post-operative ERCP).

Mortality, as mentioned previously, is very low in all approaches, and therefore is often not used as a parameter to compare different treatment options. In our series, mortality is 0.6% (3/481). All patients who died were older than 75 years, were within the first 100 patients of the series and died from medical (e.g., cardiac) rather than surgical complications (e.g., bile leak, pancreatitis, bleeding). ERCP itself also has recognised mortality which seems to be less age-related, existing even in the young-age group [36]. It is likely that our case selection for LBDE has become more rigorous after the first 100 patients. We now recommend that patients older than 75 years and/or with multiple co-morbidities may be better suited to ERCP with endoscopic sphincterotomy (ES) rather than laparoscopic cholecystectomy with LBDE [1], but clearly final decision making is made on a case-by-case basis.

Closure After Accessing the CBD

In LBDE, unlike ERCP, an anterograde approach to the bile duct is required, which can be achieved through a choledochotomy in the more traditional transductal approach, or through the more innovative transcystic route. The former generally offers easier access to the CBD (for both proximal and distal choledochoscopy), allows retrieval of larger stones and generally requires less deflection of the choledochoscope (therefore arguably less operator skill). All of these advantages pale into insignificance when it comes to its closure. In 1985, Brian Ashby knew that primary closure of the CBD should only be performed when the ampulla was shown to be open during choledochoscopy [28]. Therefore, the most common practice since the work of Professor Hans Kehr in the early twentieth century was closure of the bile duct over a T-tube. In the following sections, the different ways in which the CBD can be closed after choledochotomy are discussed: T-tube, antegrade stent, and primary closure with and without transcystic drainage.

T-Tube vs Antegrade Stent

After a choledochotomy, the CBD has traditionally been closed over a T-tube, and this is the practice that was adopted in 1998 when our institutional experience of LBDE was born. However, it was soon realised that this method was not exempt of complications. After instrumentation within the CBD that is required for the extraction of stones, papillary oedema may develop thus leading to a pressure increase inside of the CBD [37]. Therefore, since the work of Kehr, the CBD has been closed after being decompressed by a T-tube [38]. As demonstrated by Ashby in 1985, there has always been underlying interest in primary closure of choledochotomy, and he reported an undetermined number of cases with bile in the intra-operatively placed abdominal drain. Despite that, he emphasized that an hermetic closure of the duct had been achieved and that he used 3-0 catgut for the said closure [28]. The T-tube also has a secondary function besides decompressing the biliary tree and affords percutaneous access to the bile duct in the event of retained stones [39]. Laparoscopic insertion of a T-tube is associated with a 6–30% complication rate which is similar to data following open surgery [40]. Furthermore, T-tubes are uncomfortable, can be painful for patients, delay patient's return to work and have a negative impact on quality of life. There is also a risk of accidental removal/dislodgement resulting in bile leakage and biliary peritonitis [40, 41].

A retrospective study from 2002 reported a T-tube related complications in 15% of patients [42]. At that time, our institutional complication rate associated with T-tube closure of choledochotomy was 8.7% and therefore an alternative method was proposed: closure of the bile duct over an anterograde stent [43]. In 2003, after incorporating this technique into our practice, we compared the outcomes from both types of closures: T-tube vs anterograde stent [40, 44]. At that time, the series contained 61 patients and after excluding eight transcystic explorations, the remaining 53 patients were analysed. Thirty-two patients underwent closure of choledochotomy with T-tube and 21 over an anterograde stent. Amongst the complications associated with T-tube insertion that had been described: dislodgement and obstruction [45], bile leak [46], duodenal erosion [47], skin problems and ascending cholangitis [48, 49], we had already seen most of them during our early experience. In the stented group, although 10% of patients presented with hyperamylasaemia, the encouraging finding was that there were no bile leaks, and they had shorter hospital stay. There appeared to be better outcomes in favour of stented choledochorraphy. With these results and based on the available evidence at the time [50–52], this method became the standard closure after choledochotomy [40].

Some 5 years later in 2008, we published the largest known consecutive series of stented choledochorraphy after LBDE (n = 140; closure over stent = 70) [44]. Stent related complications included eight (11.2%) patients with hyperamylasaemia, with only two (2.8%) patients fulfilling Atlanta criteria for acute pancreatitis. One (1.4%) patient presented with an upper GI bleed from duodenal erosion secondary to the stent (Fig. 7.3), which was treated endoscopically with adrenaline

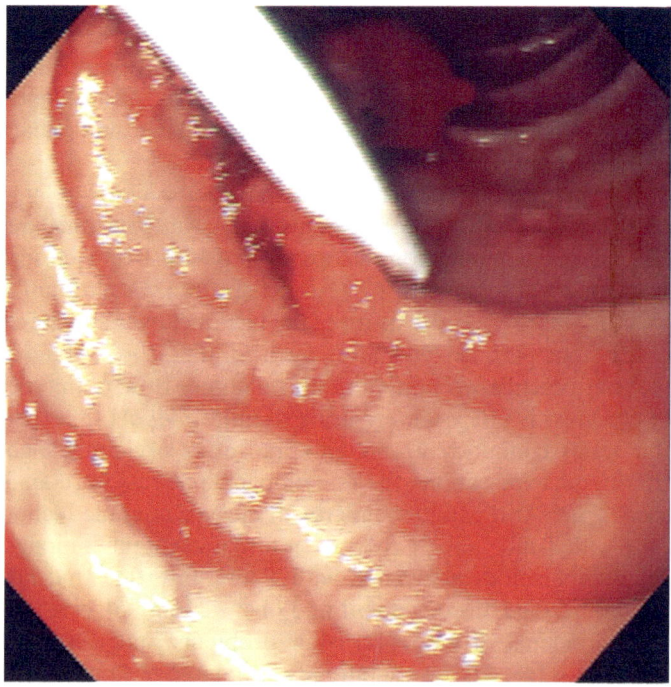

FIGURE 7.3 Stent related bleeding

injection and stent removal. One (1.4%) patient died and the median hospital stay was 4 days [2]. Spurred on by these outcomes, the technique was continued until our next institutional review of 206 patients in 2012 [53]. This contemporary analysis discovered a high incidence of stent-related pancreatitis that demanded a stop to its routine use in favour of primary closure. Transductal access was performed in 88.5% patients and in 133 patients the CBD was closed over a stent. A biochemical hyperamylasaemia was observed in 26% of those patients, however, acute pancreatitis was diagnosed in 12% of patients in accordance with Atlanta criteria [54]. Although the sample size was small, we noticed that patients managed with stented choledochorraphy who underwent prior ERCP-ES had a much lower incidence of acute pancreatitis (3.4%). It is possible that a history of sphincterotomy may be protective against acute pancreatitis in those patients who undergo closure of choledochotomy with an anterograde stent [5, 44].

Primary Closure

Following the high incidence of acute pancreatitis associated with stented choledochorraphy, primary closure of choledochotomy was then adopted and continues to be the current standard. If there are any doubts regarding biliary drainage or the patency of the papilla, we choose to protect the closure by decompressing the bile duct with a transcystic drain.

A meta-analysis of 956 patients who underwent LBDE comparing choledochotomy closure with and without a T-tube found that the former presented with more postoperative complications [55]. The study concluded that CBD drainage should be reserved for special cases. This is further supported by randomised studies that have demonstrated primary closure as the preferred method after transductal exploration [55–57]. The authors reported it to be safe and subject to less complications when compared to closure with a T-tube. In our experience, bile leak occurred in 14% of patients who underwent primary closure, however, only 4% required intervention with the remaining 10% having a mild grade A bile leak [58]. In our current practice, when a choledochotomy is performed (~10% cases) in the absence of papillary stenosis, we favour primary closure [2]. The use of a transcystic drain is reserved for high-risk patients and the T-tube for very special cases.

After completing primary closure following choledochotomy, a small leak around the sutures may occasionally be observed (Figs. 7.4 and 7.5). It is important to try to assess what extent this might be clinically relevant and decide when to reopen the choledochotomy and decompress the bile duct with a T-tube (or anterograde stent in rare instances) or insert a transcystic drain to prevent a bile leak. However, it is not always straightforward and consistently predictable. Figure 7.4 shows a primary closure following transductal exploration in a patient with previous cholecystectomy, precluding the use

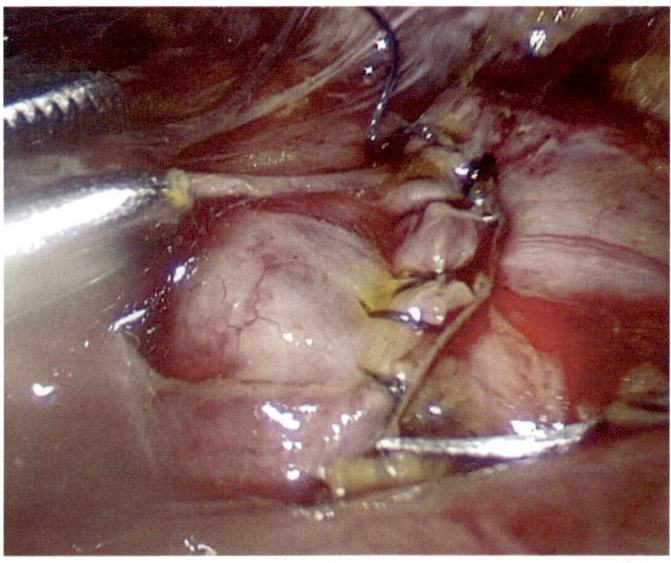

FIGURE 7.4 Primary closure with intra-operative signs of impending bile leak

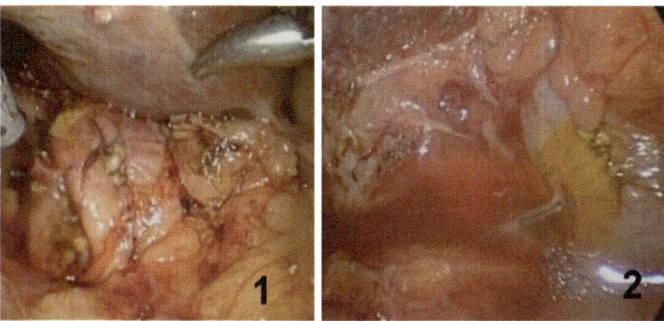

FIGURE 7.5 Primary closure of choledochotomy (1). closure with no leak (2). closure with a leak

of the preferred transcystic route for LBDE. The procedure was complex for two reasons; firstly, multiple pre-operative ERCPs had failed to clear the duct and secondly, (as predicted by the ABCdE score—see Chap. 5, section "Which patients might require LABEL?") a complex and lengthy LABEL procedure was required due to a large impacted stone. As seen in the figure, there is a tint of bile around the needle entries of the sutures. This was not appreciated intra-operatively and assessed appropriately. Post-operatively, the patient developed a grade C leak that required re-laparoscopy and subsequent ERCP with insertion of a covered metal stent. In hindsight and after reflection, the choledochotomy should have been reopened and closed over a T-tube or perhaps over an anterograde stent (the previous ERCP-ES would have rendered the patient low-risk for stent-induced pancreatitis) [44]. Note that a transcystic drain would not have been possible due to the previous cholecystectomy. Conversely, Fig. 7.5 (1) shows primary close without any intra-operative signs of bile leakage, however, the patient presented 24 h later with biliary peritonitis and required laparoscopy with T-tube insertion for a grade C bile leak. The patient in Fig. 7.5 (2), which demonstrates primary closure with signs of bile leakage, had an uneventful post-operative recovery with removal of the drain (which did not procedure any bile) on the first post-operative day. Assessing the adequacy of primary closure to predict whether a clinically significant bile leak will develop based on the intra-operative appearance of the closure is very difficult. Bile leak constitutes the Achilles heel of bile duct exploration, and without doubt, the transductal approach is the main source of it. Therefore, use of the transductal approach should be minimised to 'special' unavoidable situations. When a choledochotomy is performed, and after ensuring patency of the papilla, a very delicate technique for its closure will be required using a 5–0 absorbable suture on a small round bodied needle [2]. If an ensuing bile leak is suspected after primary closure, the surgeon should not hesitate to reopen the choledochorraphy and decompress it with an antegrade stent, T-tube or transcystic drain. Recently, an article reported the use of fibrin-collagen to protect the choledochorraphy [59]; however, we believe that the best strategy to avoid a bile leak should not be to use an adjunct for the closure of the choledochotomy, but to minimise the number of choledochotomies performed altogether [60]. Afterall, prevention is better than a cure!

Achieving Higher Rates of Transcystic LBDE: Leveraging Access to Technology and Enhanced Surgical Technique (LATEST)

Four factors have been mainly responsible for achieving higher rates of transcystic LBDE at our institution [2]. Firstly, we completely mobilise the gallbladder from the liver bed and correct the cystic duct-common bile duct junction so that the cystic duct is perpendicular to the CBD. This allows for easier cystic duct intubation, even in challenging cases (see Chap. 4, sections "Cholecystectomy" and "Intra-operative cholangiogram (IOC)"), and transcystic choledochoscopy both distally (towards the duodenum) and proximally (towards the liver). Secondly, liberal use of ultra-thin (~3 mm) choledochoscopes (at our institution we prefer disposable scopes) allows transcystic LBDE even in the presence of a thin cystic duct. Thirdly, the use of lithotripsy (the LABEL procedure—see Chap. 5) allows transcystic stone extraction even for large and/or impacted CBD stones [23–25]. Fourthly, the trans-infundibular approach (TIA) permits transcystic LBDE even when there is severe inflammation within Calot's triangle [61].

Figure 7.6 shows the total number of cases performed per year since 1998 until 2020 (**red**), along with total number of transcystic explorations (**blue**) and the % of cases performed transcystically (**black**). There is a sharp increase in the percentage of transcystic explorations after 2014 which coincides with the *'Leveraging Access to Technology and Enhanced Surgical Technique'* (LATEST) era [27]. It is through this process that we have been able to maximise the transcystic exploration rate which forms a key component of what we later defined as the *'Biliary Surgery 2.0'* concept (Fig. 7.7) [26].

3 mm Choledochoscopes

Since the first choledochoscopy in the UK by Longland in 1975 [62], the quality and availability of devices have substan-

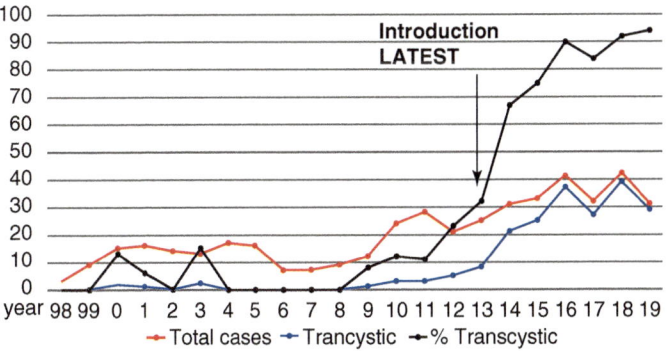

FIGURE 7.6 LBDE cases 1998–2019. Total number of cases (red), transcystic (blue) and % transcystic (black)

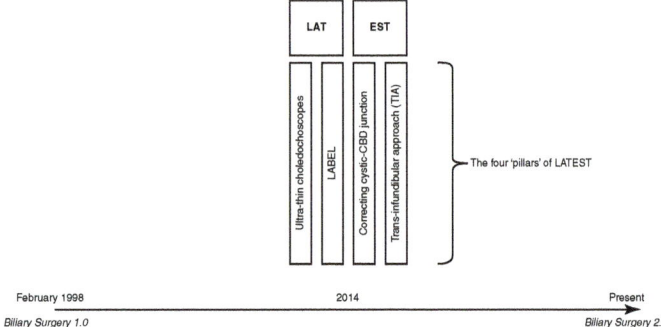

FIGURE 7.7 The four 'pillars' of Leveraging Access to Technology and Enhanced Surgical Technique (LATEST) to increase the rate of transcystic LBDE and its contribution as a key component towards the 'Biliary Surgery 2.0' concept

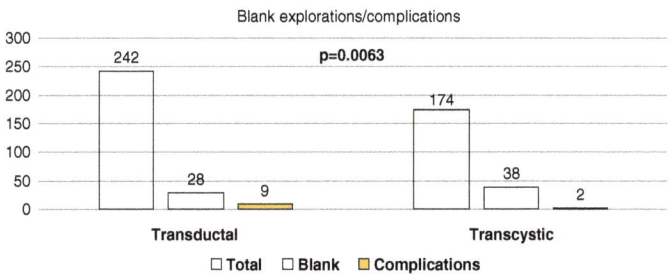

FIGURE 7.8 Incidence of negative (blank) choledochoscopy and its related morbidity for both transductal and transcystic LBDE

tially improved. The use of 3 mm ultra-thin choledochoscopes allows access to the CBD through a non-dilated cystic duct with minimal morbidity (Fig. 7.8). Currently, the available choledochoscopes are fibreoptic or digital, of which the latter can be either reusable or disposable (see Chap. 4, section "Choledochoscopes").

In our experience, we prefer to use disposable choledochoscopes. Firstly, the image quality is superior compared to the reusable fibreoptic, and secondly, we believe it to be more cost effective. The cost of initial purchase plus maintenance, repairs and sterilization of reusable choledochoscopes is likely to be more than using disposable 3 mm choledochoscopes. Furthermore, if reusable instruments were preferred, at least three functioning choledochoscopes would be needed in order to be able to offer a reliable service. This would be the minimum requirement and allow for one on the shelf, one sent for sterilization (that very often occurs elsewhere offsite) and one which may have been sent for repairs (the 3 mm reusable choledochoscopes are very easily damaged through improper handling).

Between February 1998 and February 2020 (prior to the effect of the SARS-CoV-2 global pandemic on the UK) we had performed 460 LBDEs at our institution. In the pre-LATEST era (prior to February 2014), which we refer to as *'Biliary Surgery 1.0'*, 237 explorations had been undertaken whereas 223 were carried out after February 2014 (LATEST era). During the pre-LATEST era only 11% CBD explorations were accessed through the transcystic route compared to 85% during the LATEST era. Ultra-thin 3 mm choledochoscopes have been increasingly used at our institution and during recent times have been the scope diameter of choice. In the pre-LATEST era, we had not used 3 mm choledochoscopes at all (the 11% transcystic explorations were all performed with 5 mm choledochoscopes), however, since the introduction of LATEST, 3 mm choledochoscopy was performed in 35% of patients (41% of transcystic explorations). In the last 50 patients this had increased to 90% of patients and 90% of transcystic explorations. We hypothesise that the 11% of transcystic explorations performed with a 5 mm choledochoscope prior to February 2014 was only possible because the cystic duct was dilated and accommodated a larger diameter scope. It is reasonable to assume that the majority of the remaining cases did not have a dilated cystic duct and therefore the non-availability of a 3 mm choledochoscope would have been a major factor that precluded transcystic exploration prior to February 2104 (pre-LATEST era). As previously mentioned, we favour disposable, single-use choledochoscopes and the recently launched SpyGlass™

Discover (9F with external diameter 3 mm) by Boston Scientific is a good example and is currently the only choledochoscope on the market with 4-way steering (see Table 4.2). PUSEN Medical Technology Co® just released their thinnest choledochoscope to date with an external diameter of 2.5 mm (equivalent to 7.5F) which will allow intubation of even narrower cystic ducts. Routine use of ~3 mm choledochoscopes not only increased the overall transcystic exploration rate, but also increased the number of negative (blank) examinations, which was not associated with increased morbidity (Fig. 7.8). There were only two post-operative complications from 38 negative transcystic choledochoscopies [2]. Moreover, the number of negative (blank) choledochoscopies was not greatly influenced by whether or not we performed an intra-operative cholangiogram (IOC), and our threshold to perform choledochoscopy lowered as procedural experience increased. This should not be surprising, because at the beginning of the series, a choledochotomy would have been necessary to perform choledochoscopy. During the first (chronological) quartile (n = 120), the negative choledochoscopy rate was 18%, which rose to 34% (almost double) during the last quartile of the series (p = 0.0077) [2] (Fig. 7.2). To summarise, our current practice is to perform transcystic choledochoscopy in patients with an abnormal or equivocal IOC, patients with allergy to radiological contrast or pregnant patients [2]. Although, a very valid alternative in these patients is to perform laparoscopic intra-operative ultrasound (LIOUS—see Chap. 3).

Lithotripsy-Assisted Bile Duct Exploration by Laparoendoscopy (LABEL)

The LABEL technique has been fully described elsewhere in this book (see Chap. 5). In 2017, we published our early institutional experience of LABEL using holmium laser lithotripsy (HLL) [24]. At that time, the 'L' from LABEL stood for 'Laser', however, more recently we have expanded the definition to include all forms of lithotripsy. In 2019, we demonstrated that the use of lithotripsy techniques alone had increased our rate of successful transcystic LBDE to over 80% [23]. At the time of writing this book, our contemporary rate of successful transcystic exploration was 93% (Fig. 7.6), which has resulted from the culmination of all the factors described in section "Achieving higher rates of transcystic LBDE: Leveraging Access to Technology and Enhanced Surgical Technique (LATEST)". The LABEL technique forms one of the pillars of LATEST (Fig. 7.7). Prior to the LATEST era, LABEL was not available at our institution and the transcystic route was used in just 11% of patients. Since LATEST was introduced, LABEL was used in almost one-fifth of patients (19%) and the transcystic exploration rate increased to 85%. The surgical team should anticipate having to use LABEL at least once every five patients if there is an aspiration to achieve a near-complete transcystic LBDE practice.

Trans-Infundibular Approach (TIA) to the Bile Duct

It is well known that the transcystic approach during LBDE is associated with less complications, mainly bile leak, but for this method to be feasible, the cystic duct must be accessible in a standard or modified manner [2, 63, 64]. Transcystic access to the bile duct may be compromised when there is severe inflammation and/or fibrosis within the hepatic hilum, precluding safe dissection of Calot's triangle. There are also almost always accompanying changes to the CBD along with the inflammation and fibrosis seen at the hilum. The CBD is often inflamed and thick-walled, making choledochotomy fraught with increased risk. In this scenario, the procedure may be abandoned altogether, the operation completed with a subtotal cholecystectomy and/or converted to open surgery. The presence of CBD stones would also mandate a postoperative ERCP to clear the bile duct [65–68]. In 2018, we published a series of patients who underwent LBDE despite the intra-operative finding of a 'frozen' hilum due to severe inflammation and fibrosis [61]. Access to the bile duct was achieved via a trans-infundibular approach (TIA) as conventional access to the cystic duct was denied, however, this approach still qualifies as a transcystic LBDE. Our first experience of performing this technique was coincidentally also our first reported use of the LABEL procedure in February 2014. TIA forms another pillar of LATEST and specifically pertains to '*Enhanced Surgical Technique*' (Fig. 7.7). We have only used the TIA technique during the LATEST era, and within this time, it has been required in 13 of 244 (5.3%) patients who have undergone LBDE at our institution. Therefore, one in 20 patients undergoing acute biliary surgery for complex gallstone disease within our series had a frozen hilum, and without the TIA to the bile duct, we would have failed transcystic LBDE in approximately 5% of our patients during the LATEST era. Failure of transcystic LBDE in this subgroup of patients is perhaps more clinically significant, as often a choledochotomy cannot or should not be performed, with subtotal cholecystectomy and post-operative ERCP being one of the only remaining feasible (but unsatisfactory) options left.

The TIA to the bile duct is not completely new. Chen et al., described a novel method of transcystic choledochoscopy by introducing the choledochoscope through the gallbladder fundus [69]. However, the objective of their technique was not to overcome the hazardous dissection of a hostile, frozen Calot's triangle, but instead their aim was to demonstrate a technique that avoided the difficulty of laparoscopic intubation of the cystic duct with a choledochoscope. The author's initial report of this technique resulted in successful transcystic CBD clearance in just 78% of patients. The reasons for failure included a narrow cystic duct and unfavourable anatomy of the cystic duct-common bile duct junction. As already extensively described, for routine cases with a permissible hepatic hilum, we advocate complete mobilisation of the gallbladder from the liver bed and correction of the cystic duct-common bile duct junction so that the cystic duct is perpendicular to the CBD (see Chap. 4, section "Cholecystectomy"). The correction of this cystic angle enables cannulation of the cystic duct for IOC and facilitates intubation of the cystic duct for transcystic choledochoscopy [2]. We only advocate using the TIA-LBDE technique to overcome the challenging scenario of severe inflammation and/or fibrosis within Calot's triangle rather than achieving transcystic choledochoscopy in cases where the cystic duct can be accessed in the traditional manner [61, 70]. The TIA technique can also be useful in obtaining an IOC in situations where the cystic duct cannot be clearly identified and therefore cannulated. Figure 7.9 demonstrates TIA-choledochoscopy in a patient with a frozen hepatic hilum (left image). Contrast was then injected through the working channel of the choledochoscope to obtain a cholangiogram (TIA-cholangiogram) (right image). In this scenario, a cholangiogram can be extremely useful in enabling the surgeon to orientate themselves with the cystic and common duct anatomy and therefore facilitate further 'safe' dissection of a frozen Calot's triangle. If a subtotal cholecystectomy is unavoidable, TIA can be useful in excluding stones within the remnant gallbladder as it is important to ensure that the infundibulum is free of stones.

Once the CBD has been cleared, the infundibulum will need to be closed primarily. The severe inflammation and fibrosis within the hepatic hilum can draw the CBD towards the infundibulum. The possibility of closing the infundibulum with resulting stenosis of the bile duct should be strongly considered after using the TIA technique. Therefore, in this scenario, we have chosen to close the infundibulum with a disposable choledochoscope inside of the CBD to protect it from stenosis, which is then removed after the penultimate suture (Fig. 7.10).

At the time of publishing our series of trans-infundibular choledochoscopy, about half of the patients required a joint TIA-LABEL technique [61]. The TIA technique can be further enhanced by combining this approach with lithotripsy, especially for patients with type II Mirizzi syndrome or a

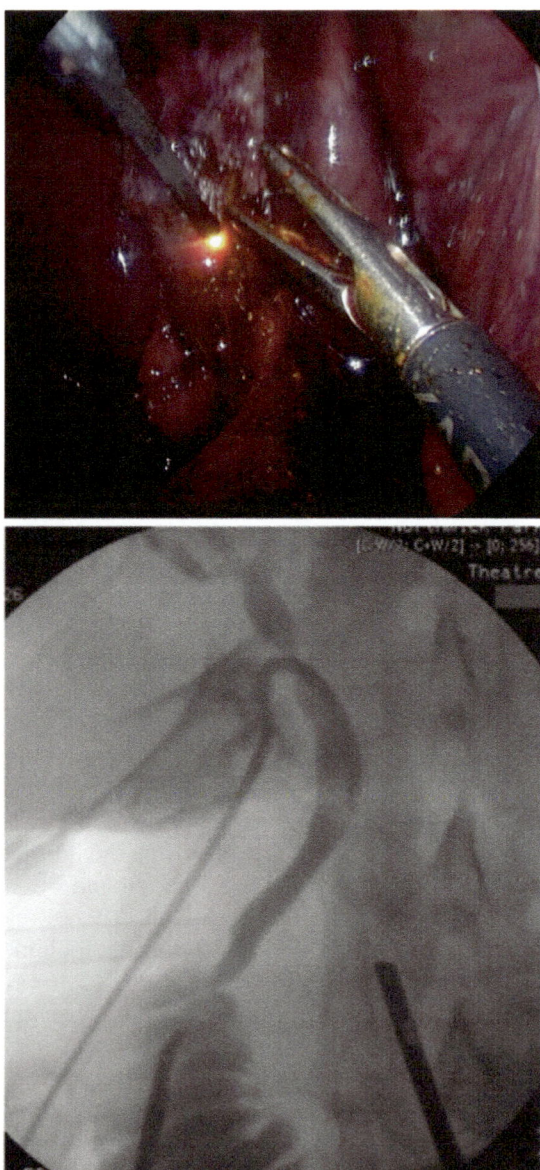

FIGURE 7.9 Trans-infundibular approach (TIA)-cholangiogram obtained through the working channel of the choledochoscope

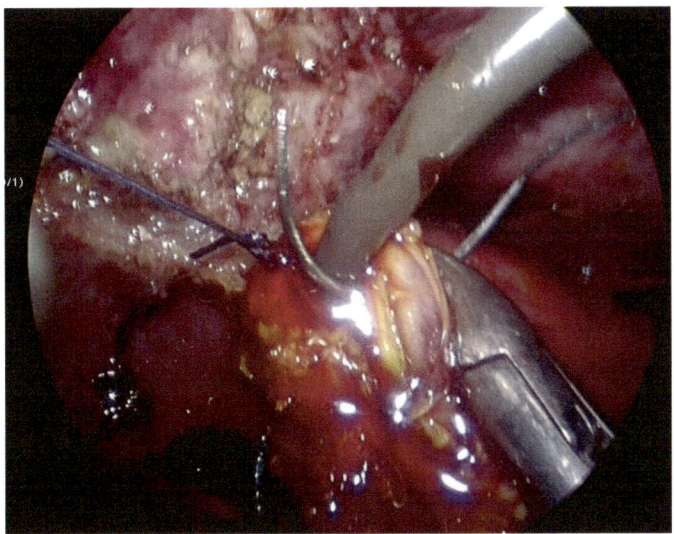

FIGURE 7.10 Closure of the infundibulum following the TIA technique with a choledochoscope inserted into CBD

large impacted stone. This is perhaps not surprising as we suspect that many of the patients who had a 'frozen' (impossible) hepatic hilum most likely had Mirizzi syndrome (and probably type II). Prior to the establishment of LABEL, these cases would have either resulted in failure of stone clearance or necessitated choledochotomy. In cases of severe inflammation and/or fibrosis within Calot's triangle, choledochotomy is best avoided due to the hostile environment and questionable integrity of the bile duct wall, which would result in an increased risk of bile leak. Avoiding choledochotomy, especially in such cases, should be the primary aim. Having said that, there may be extremely rare circumstances where it is unavoidable, and the TIA technique can assist in siting the appropriate location of the choledochotomy within a frozen hilum. This can be achieved by transilluminating through the bile duct wall from its lumen using the light source from the choledochoscope introduced via TIA. This scenario was encountered when in one patient we found that the angle of deflection of the choledochoscope inserted via TIA was suboptimal to perform the LABEL technique of an impacted intra-hepatic stone. This procedure was completed prior to the availability of the newer ultra-thin 4-way steering choledochoscopes (SpyGlass™ Discover) which may have overcome this issue. Trans-infundibular choledochoscopy was used to transilluminate the safe position for choledochotomy in an inflamed duct [61]. This particular patient had a successful transductal stone extraction and subsequently an uneventful recovery without complication. Open and laparoscopic subtotal cholecystectomy are considered as feasible operative techniques when variable anatomy or other intra-operative findings preclude safe dissection of Calot's triangle. Surgery performed in a patient with a 'frozen' hilum often ends in subtotal cholecystectomy, however, these patients also represent a high-risk population for choledocholithiasis. In 2015, a meta-analysis reported outcomes from subtotal cholecystectomy from 30 studies (1231 patients) [66]. In this study, severe cholecystitis, inflammation and fibrosis within Calot's triangle was the indication for subtotal cholecystectomy in nearly three quarters of the patients. The authors found that 3.1% of patients who underwent subtotal cholecystectomy subsequently presented with symptomatic retained stones. Of those, 13.2% and 78.9% underwent subsequent LBDE and post-operative ERCP respectively. TIA cholangiography with choledochoscopy can help the surgeon to clarify distorted or variable anatomy in these cases thereby facilitating complete dissection of the vital structures within Calot's triangle and the safe completion of a total cholecystectomy together with successful CBD clearance when indicated.

Transcystic Vs Transductal Access

The updated guidelines for the management of choledocholithiasis from the British Society of Gastroenterology (BSG) reports a lack of evidence for superiority in efficacy, morbidity or mortality between LBDE and perioperative ERCP [71]. In keeping with such guidelines, several studies (systematic reviews and randomised trials) have failed to demonstrate significant difference in morbidity following one-stage (laparoscopic cholecystectomy + LBDE) and two-stage (preoperative ERCP followed by laparoscopic cholecystectomy) management of CBD stones with concomitant gallstones (see Table 2.2). In a meta-analysis by Ricci et al., 915 patients from 14 randomised controlled trials (RCTs) who underwent LBDE were included [72]. However, *transcystic* LBDE was only performed in about a third of these patients (36.2%), and therefore almost two-thirds were subject to transductal exploration via choledochotomy. This has been confirmed in our own analysis of 23 RCTs published within the last two decades, and from the 16 studies published in English, the transcystic approach was attempted in just 32% (305/953) of patients (Table 2.4) [73]. As previously discussed in Chap. 2, section "Bile leak", the morbidity of LBDE is primarily represented by bile leak (if a choledochotomy is performed and closed primarily or with a T-tube) and secondarily by pancreatitis (if a choledochotomy is performed and closed over an antegrade stent). In studies with a high rate of transductal LBDE, the reported rates of bile leak have been as high as 13.3–16.7% [16, 63]. Liu et al., reported that the total incidences of bile leakage in the laparoscopic and endoscopic groups from eight studies included in their systematic review were 6.3% and 0.5% respectively [33]. Two meta-analyses have further proven that transcystic, when compared to transductal LBDE, resulted in significantly less bile leaks and overall morbidity, shorter operative time and hospital stay, reduced operative blood loss, and reduced costs (increased cost efficiency) [34, 35]. Post-procedure acute pancreatitis occurs more frequently in patients who undergo endoscopic management of their CBD stones compared to patients who undergo LBDE [4, 72]. It should be noted that this difference is still appreciated despite many of the randomised trials having contained many patients within the LBDE arm who had closure of choledochotomy over an antegrade stent [74–77]. The link between antegrade stenting and acute pancreatitis is thought to be due to instrumentation of the biliary sphincter [78]. Our earlier institutional data demonstrated an incidence of acute pancreatitis in 12% (and 26% hyperamylasaemia) of patients following closure of choledochotomy over an antegrade stent [53]. In 2020, we reported our outcomes from 416 consecutive LBDEs and demonstrated that transcystic LBDE resulted in significantly lower major (Clavien-Dindo III-IV) and minor (Clavien-Dindo I-II) morbidity when compared to transductal LBDE (1.1% vs 5.8%, p = 0.0181 and 8.0% vs 21.9%, p = 0.0001 respectively) [2]. In particular, bile leak was significantly reduced (1.1% vs 5.8%, p = 0.0181) as well as post-procedural pancreatitis (0.6% vs 7.4%, p = 0.0005). When approximately only a third of patients who underwent LBDE during prospective randomised trials received a transcystic approach, the pooled morbidity associated with bile leak from LBDE is certainly an over-estimate of the true morbidity associated with a contemporary transcystic predominant (>80–90%) LBDE practice. We have noted just one patient with a bile leak from our last 100 patients (1%) from our transcystic predominant (>90%) LBDE practice (Table 7.1). Furthermore, with higher rates of transcystic exploration, the morbidity associated with acute pancreatitis (secondary to closure of choledochotomy over an antegrade stent) would also be lower than that currently reported in the literature. From our last 100 patients who underwent LBDE, the incidence of post-procedural acute pancreatitis has been zero (Table 7.1). Currently, evidence to evaluate the outcomes of laparoscopic cholecystectomy with transcystic LBDE alone versus laparoscopic cholecystectomy with pre-, intra- or post operative ERCP is lacking and further studies in this area should be a focus of future research.

There is a learning curve associated with the transcystic approach. In particular, since 2014 we have experienced an increase in the rate of transcystic explorations following the adoption of ultra-thin choledochoscopes at our centre and the introduction of LABEL and TIA techniques (see section "Achieving higher rates of transcystic LBDE: Leveraging Access to Technology and Enhanced Surgical Technique (LATEST)"). These landmark changes to our practice have been embodied in what we have termed 'LATEST' in LBDE and enabled a >90% transcystic exploration rate from our last 100 consecutive LBDE patients. Moreover, unpublished data from a surgeon at an institution outside of the UK, who received our mentoring, has achieved similar rates of transcystic exploration in their first 100 procedures. This suggests that it is not only the learning curve, but also applying the LATEST principles coupled with mentoring that can result in similar outcomes to the last 100 procedures from our series, which have been performed after two decades of experience in LBDE! The advantage of the transcystic approach is that it is not necessary to close the common duct, and as described in great detail, closure after choledochotomy is the main source of post-operative morbidity. Mastering the transcystic approach is technically demanding and requires incorporating all four pillars of LATEST into routine practice (Fig. 7.7). Without ultra-thin choledochoscopes and LABEL, the basket-in-catheter (BIC) technique can be used to achieve transcystic exploration [79]. Although our preference is for exploration under direct vision using choledochoscopy, rather than exploration under fluoroscopic guidance, we have used this technique successfully on three occasions in patients with narrow cystic and common ducts when a 3 mm choledochoscope was not available. The group who described the BIC technique, increased their transcystic exploration rate from 55% to 70% [79]. As previously mentioned, exploring the CBD via the transcystic route lowers the threshold to perform choledochoscopy in patients who are pregnant, have a contrast allergy or have an equivocal IOC. A low threshold for transcystic choledochoscopy is another significant advantage of transcystic LBDE. Figure 7.11 summarises our institutional algorithm for the surgical management of proven or suspected choledocholithiasis with concomitant gallstones.

In 2019, Hajibandeh et al., published the most recent systematic review comparing transcystic and transductal LBDE and included 4073 patients from 30 studies [80]. The authors found that there was no difference in CBD clearance rates, however, and reported lower overall complications, biliary complications, blood loss and reduced length of stay with the transcystic approach. The findings were congruent with our own institutional data and the previously described systematic

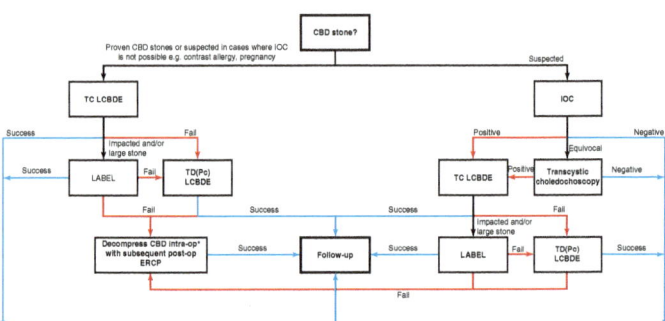

FIGURE 7.11 Management algorithm for proven or suspected cho-ledocholithiasis. *Placing a common bile duct stent and/or inserting a T-tube and/or placing transcystic drain. *CBD* common bile duct, *TC* transcystic, *TD* transductal, *Pc* primary closure, *LCBDE* laparo-scopic common bile duct exploration, *IOC* intra-operative cholangiogram, *LABEL* lithotripsy-assisted bile duct exploration by laparoendoscopy, *ERCP* endoscopic retrograde cholangiopancreatography

reviews [2, 34, 35]. From the 30 studies included in their meta-analysis, 10 were prospective and 20 were retrospective observational studies. The two largest individual studies, were by Paganini et al. (retrospective study with 329 patients) [78] and Zhang et al. (prospective study with 330 patients) [81]. Our study from 2020, albeit retrospective in nature, represents the largest single study to date comparing outcomes from transcystic and transductal LBDE [2].

Management of Type II Mirizzi Syndrome

In 2020, we reported our outcomes from 11 patients following the laparoscopic management of type II Mirizzi syndrome [70]. Mirizzi syndrome is an uncommon complication of long-standing gallstone disease. It was first described by Kehr in 1905 and Ruge in 1908, as a rare form of obstructive jaundice caused by external obstruction of the bile duct by an impacted stone in the cystic duct with associated inflammation [82].

However, the eponymous accreditation was given to Pablo Mirizzi in 1948 who defined the condition as compression of the hepatic duct by an impacted gallstone in the cystic duct or gallbladder neck. Compression of an impacted gallstone leads to pressure ulceration with subsequent local inflammation, resulting first in external compression (obstruction) of the bile duct then further erosion into the bile duct. An evolving cholecystocholedochal fistula will ensue with varying degrees of communication between the gallbladder and bile duct (Fig. 7.12) [83, 84].

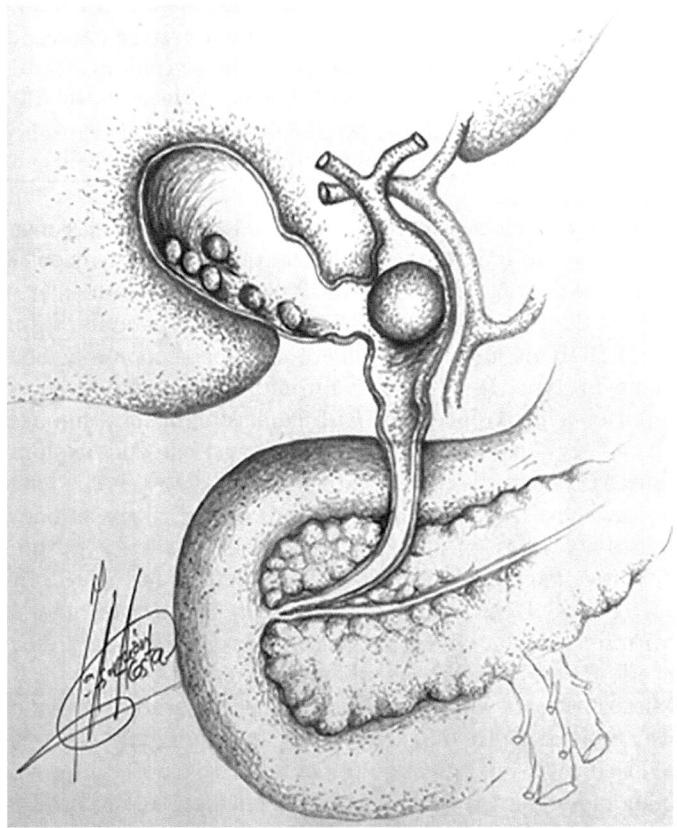

FIGURE 7.12 Type II Mirizzi syndrome

There have been several classifications of this complex disease since its description, but only two are in wide use. McSherry classified Mirizzi syndrome into types based on ERCP findings [85]. Type I was characterised by the extrinsic compression of the common hepatic duct (CHD) or proximal CBD due to an impacted gallstone in the infundibulum or cystic duct with subsequent inflammation. Type II was defined by its association with a cholecystocholedochal fistula. Csendes' classification further divided the communication between the gallbladder and bile duct into three types depending on the size of the fistula in relation to the circumference of the CBD (Csendes' I being equivalent to McSherry I, and Csendes' II, III and IV involving less than one-third, between one-third and two-thirds, and more than two-thirds of the circumference of the CBD respectively) [82]. In 2007, Csendes' classification was extended to include the presence of a cholecystoenteric fistula together with any other form of Mirizzi (Csendes' V) [86]. Our series of type II Mirizzi syndrome has been classified according to McSherry's classification [70]. The incidence of Mirizzi syndrome appears to be higher within Asian and South American populations [87–89]. At the time of writing, 2.7% (13/481) of patients within our LBDE database had undergone laparoscopic management of type II Mirizzi syndrome. Other authors have reported a higher incidence, with similar frequencies amongst all cholecystectomies, rather than amongst bile duct explorations as in our series [90]. Pre-operative diagnosis is challenging as there are no defining symptoms or signs and low sensitivity rates of imaging tests. The sensitivity of pre-operative imaging is variable and summarised in Table 7.2 [87, 91, 92]. ERCP has the highest sensitivity for the diagnosis of Mirizzi syndrome and is considered the gold standard diagnostic tool. However, we observed that four of the type II Mirizzi patients within our series had pre-operative ERCP, of which none were diagnostic and the condition was only realised intra-operatively. Pre-operative diagnosis improves outcomes of surgery, allowing better planning and referral to an appropriate surgeon.

TABLE 7.2 Diagnostic sensitivity of pre-operative imaging for Mirizzi syndrome

Modality	Sensitivity (%)
US	8.3–27
CT	25–31
MRCP	50–63
ERCP	55–90

At present, there is no general consensus for the management of Mirizzi syndrome and in particular type II Mirizzi syndrome. The available evidence still recommends open cholecystectomy for the management of Mirizzi syndrome [89, 92]. However, some surgeons have recommended a laparoscopic approach, but only for patients with confirmed type I Mirizzi syndrome [91, 93, 94] and others have described their laparoscopic technique for patients with type II Mirizzi syndrome [95, 96]. Regarding endoscopic treatment, peroral cholangioscopy-directed lithotripsy has been reported to successfully treat complex bile duct stones in patients with Mirizzi syndrome; however, the anomalous anatomy is not corrected which might explained the high recurrence rate (16%) [91]. Finally, a combined laparoendoscopic approach for type II Mirizzi syndrome has also been described consisting of pre-operative ERCP and laparoscopic subtotal cholecystectomy [97]. In our type II Mirizzi syndrome series, laparoscopic success rate has been 100% with no conversions to open surgery, but there was a trend towards increased bile leak (18%) compared to non-Mirizzi LBDE (3.8%) (p = 0.06) [70]. Zhu et al., reported two cases of Mirizzi amongst their 14 conversions to open surgery (14%) in their series of 708 patients [3]. Kumar et al., managed to complete just one case laparoscopically from the 23 patients that they operated on [90]. The traditional approach involves access to the bile duct through a choledochotomy or fistulotomy in order to remove the stone (s) (Fig. 7.13), followed by a subtotal cholecystectomy, which leaves Hartmann's pouch to reconstruct the bile

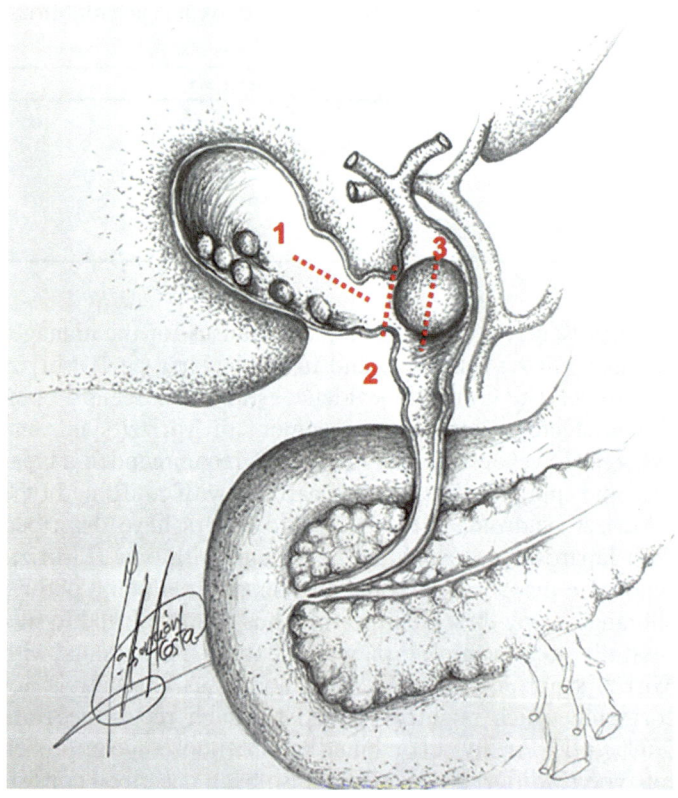

FIGURE 7.13 Incisions to access bile duct: (1) Infundibulotomy (2) Fistulotomy (3) Choledochotomy

duct over a T-tube (Figs. 7.14 and 7.15). In much larger defects, a bilioenteric anastomosis may be required [98, 99]. In some patients, we reconstructed the CBD over an indwelling stent (Fig. 7.16) whilst in others, the infundibulum was closed primarily over a 5F catheter after near-total cholecystectomy (Fig. 7.17 left and top right). The placement of the 'transcystic' drain enables a post-operative cholangiogram prior to its removal (Fig. 7.17 bottom right). The technique has evolved over the 13 cases performed since 1998. As with LBDE in general, the management of Mirizzi syndrome changed significantly since the introduction of the LABEL and TIA

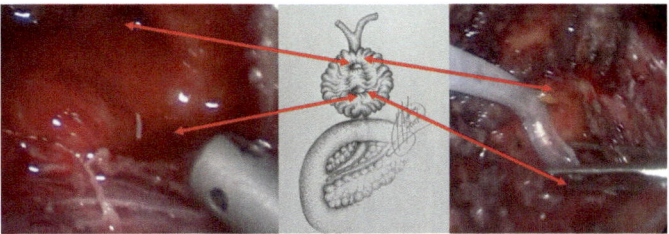

FIGURE 7.14 Type II Mirizzi syndrome: large defect with proximal and distal CBD exposed

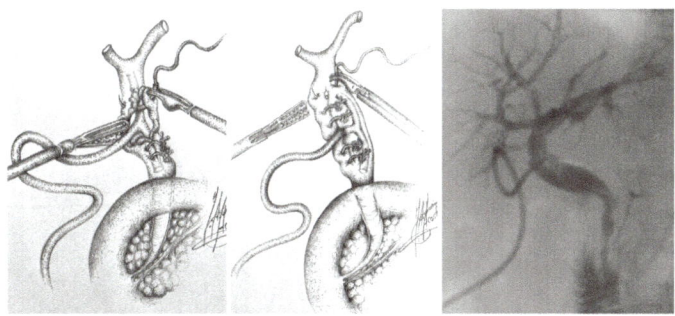

FIGURE 7.15 Repair of type II Mirizzi syndrome over a T-Tube (left and centre) and cholangiogram through the T-tube (tubogram)

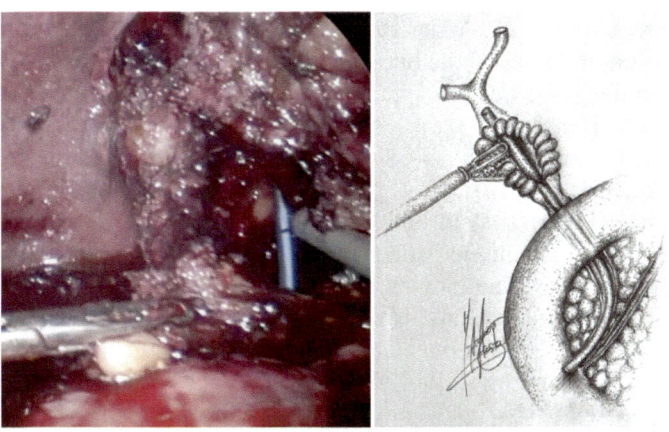

FIGURE 7.16 Type II Mirizzi syndrome: repair over an antegrade stent

236   A. Martinez-Isla et al.

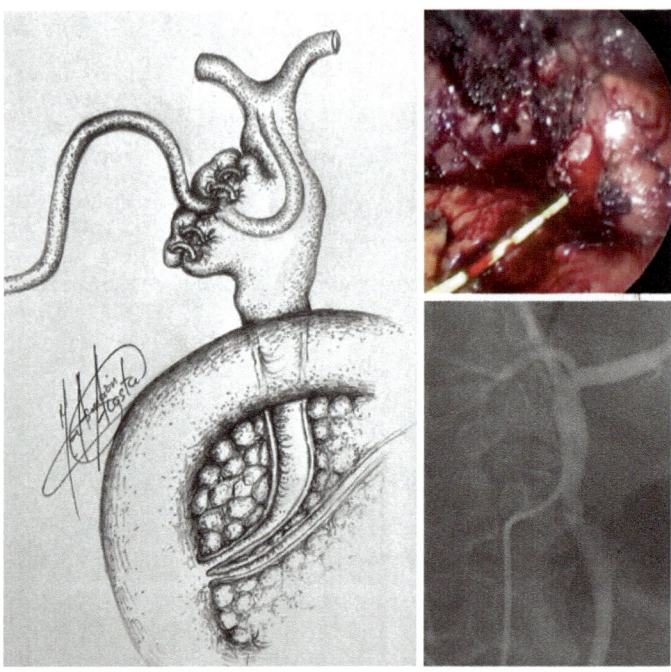

FIGURE 7.17 Type II Mirizzi síndrome: closure with transcystic drain (left and top right) and cholangiogram (bottom right)

techniques [23, 61]. The communication between the infundibulum and the bile duct in type II Mirizzi syndrome is similar to the one mentioned in our description of TIA. Therefore, TIA is a suitable adjunct to be used in type II Mirizzi syndrome (we suspect that upon hindsight, some of the early TIA-LBDEs were likely to have been undiagnosed type II Mirizzi syndrome) and can be augmented with the LABEL technique when the impacted stone cannot be removed by standard methods (Fig. 7.18). TIA for type II Mirizzi syndrome has also been described under the designation 'transfistulous bile duct exploration' (TBDE) by another group from Taiwan [96]. When we used TIA specifically for type II Mirizzi syndrome, we coined the expression 'trans-infundibulo-fistulous approach' (TIFA) [70]. TIFA enables

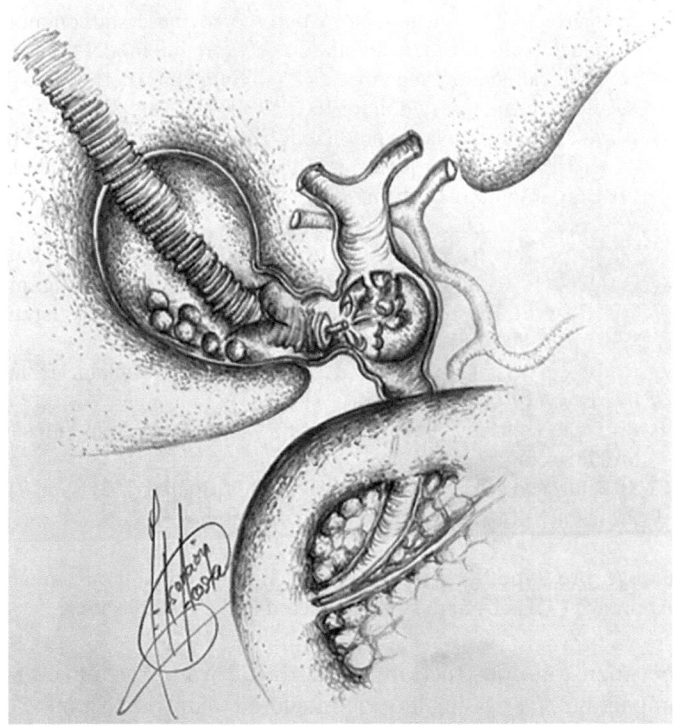

FIGURE 7.18 Type II Mirizzi syndrome: TIA-LABEL

access to the CBD from inside the gallbladder, away from the inflamed area, whilst allowing removal of impacted stones (with or without LABEL) in the area of the fistula (Fig. 7.19). It is difficult to differentiate between a dilated cystic duct in an inflamed hilum and a type II Mirizzi syndrome and can be open to interpretation. If the CBD is approached via TIA (or TIFA in type II Mirizzi syndrome), it may not be possible to make such a distinction intra-operatively. For the laparoscopic management of type II Mirizzi syndrome, we hypothesise that TIA (or TIFA) will become the standard approach. However, as discussed, if pre-operative imaging has not diagnosed type II Mirizzi syndrome, then differentiating

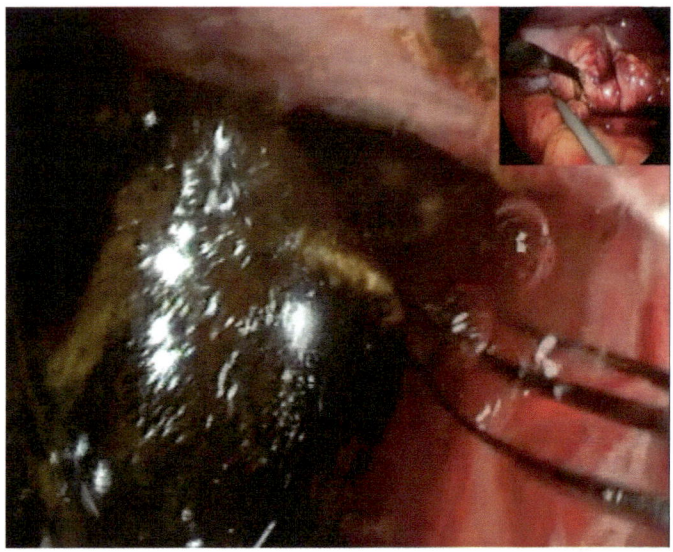

FIGURE 7.19 Type II Mirizzi syndrome: Trans-Infundibulo-Fistulous Approach (TIFA). Large stone impacted in the fistulous tract

between total destruction of the ductal wall (Fig. 7.14) and impaction of a passing large stone in the cystic duct with local inflammation of the joint cystic duct and CBD walls may not be possible intra-operatively.

The Impact of LBDE in a General Surgery Department

Emergency admissions represent up to 50% of the activity within a General Surgery department [100]. Up to one third of the emergency workload is represented by acute biliary pathology [101]. Patients with a CBD >10 mm and abnormal LFTs with an elevated bilirubin represent those at the highest risk of choledocholithiasis with an incidence of approximately 30% within this group [102]. In the UK, gallstones account for the underlying cause in about one third of patients with acute pancreatitis [103]. European Association for Endoscopic Surgery (EAES) and British Society of Gastroenterology (BSG) guidelines recommend imaging (± clearance) of the bile duct and cholecystectomy within the index admission for patients with acute gallstone pancreatitis [104, 105]. Therefore, magnetic resonance cholangiopancreatography (MRCP) ± pre-operative ERCP followed by laparoscopic cholecystectomy (two-stage management) or laparoscopic cholecystectomy + IOC ± LBDE (single-stage management) are the two most common options available within the UK [76, 105, 106]. In our practice, the aim of pre-operative imaging is simply to prove gallstones as the underlying cause, and therefore ultrasound is entirely sufficient. Patients with mild or moderate gallstone pancreatitis who are surgical candidates are offered laparoscopic cholecystectomy + IOC ± LBDE within the same admission [2]. Historical data from our institution has demonstrated the feasibility and reproducibility of single-stage laparoscopic management of acute gallstone pancreatitis [107, 108]. Adherence to current guidelines for the management of acute gallstone pancreatitis is highly variable and compliance lies between 6.6% and 89% [109–111]. At our institution, the gold standard treatment for acute gallstone pancreatitis was achieved in 66% of patients. Surgical Workload Outcomes Research Database (SWORD) is a collaborative database maintained by the Association of Upper GI Surgeons of Great Britain and Ireland (AUGIS) and the Association of Laparoscopic Surgeons of Great Britain and Ireland (ALSGBI). SWORD has reported low levels of adherence (mean 14%; range 0–40%) to the aforementioned guidelines (cholecystectomy for acute gallstone pancreatitis during the index admission or within 2 weeks of discharge) [112]. The National Confidential Enquiry into Patient Outcome and Death (NCEPOD) assessed the quality of care given to patients with acute pancreatitis [113]. Their publication, '*Acute Pancreatitis: Treat the cause*' published in 2016, found that 21% of patients within the study had one or more previous episodes of acute pancreatitis, 93% of those for the same cause. Reasons for lack of compliance are multifactorial and include financial constraints, non-availability of theatre space (both restricted access to emergency theatre lists and lack of predictable access to urgent theatre lists beyond the main emergency list), lack of expertise and delayed diagnosis (e.g., gallstones not identified on ultrasound but subsequently diagnosed by outpatient MRCP). In contrast, there was 95% compliance with national guidelines at our institution for the management of choledocholithiasis in patients presenting with jaundice, deranged LFTs and/or dilated CBD on imaging.

The creation of an acute biliary pathway at our institution has enabled better adherence to national guidelines. The pathway begins with rapid assessment within the Emergency Surgery Unit (ESU) with reliable access to ultrasound imaging within 24 h of admission. Patients with gallstones and suspected CBD stones are referred via an online platform to the acute biliary pathway. Following assessment by a surgeon, suitable patients are then scheduled to a dedicated biliary list for laparoscopic cholecystectomy + IOC ± LBDE based on clinical priority. The availability of a dedicated biliary list reduces reliance on the emergency theatre and surgical expertise in LBDE negates the need for bile duct imaging with MRCP. Monkhouse et al., retrospectively reviewed 153 admissions for acute gallstone pancreatitis and estimated additional hospital costs associated with readmissions for recurrent pancreatitis or biliary pathology [114]. The authors found that instigating a dedicated fortnightly half-day theatre list for cholecystectomy after biliary pancreatitis would be cost neutral when compared to the hospital costs related to the 40 readmissions within this group. Murphy et al., successfully implemented an Acute Care Surgery (ACS) service to facilitate index cholecystectomy for gallstone pancreatitis [115]. The same authors identified that associated financial costs and economic effectiveness of such an intervention were unknown and were therefore potential barriers to its widespread adoption. In a follow-on study, the group investigated the impact of ACS services at two hospitals before and after its implementation and found that index cholecystectomy rose from 16% to 76%, with significant reduction in readmissions and a cost saving of 12.6% ($1162) per patient undergoing cholecystectomy [116]. At a busy district general hospital (600–700 acute hospital beds) with more than 100,000 A&E attendances a year, two protected theatre sessions a week (either two half-days or one full day) would be sufficient to meet national targets for the management of acute gallstone disease (gallstone pancreatitis, acute cholecystitis and choledocholithiasis).

Biliary Surgery 2.0 Concept

If you are reading this book then you are a likely proponent of the single stage management (laparoscopic cholecystectomy + IOC ± LBDE) of choledocholithiasis with concomitant gallstones. As experience in LBDE grows, emerging evidence is supporting this strategy as the treatment of choice in patients who are fit for surgery. One of the main disadvantages of LBDE is undoubtedly the morbidity associated with bile leak. We have demonstrated that bile leak is largely associated with transductal exploration via choledochotomy. It is also important to remember that LBDE and two-staged endoscopic techniques have had similar morbidity in studies, even though the pooled data from the LBDE cohort contained two-thirds of patients who underwent transductal exploration via choledochotomy. Increasing the transcystic exploration rate in LBDE will undeniably reduce the morbidity associated with this procedure and should be the primary aim of any surgeon in their LBDE learning curve.

At our institution, we have applied four principles that have directly increased transcystic LBDE to the current rate of >90%. We have named these four 'pillars' LATEST as described in section "Achieving higher rates of transcystic LBDE: Leveraging Access to Technology and Enhanced Surgical Technique (LATEST)" [27]. Modern day minimally invasive surgery for complex gallstone disease has evolved greatly over the last two decades. We have described this progression as '*Biliary Surgery 2.0*' [26]. *Biliary Surgery 1.0* consisted of mainly transductal exploration, using 5 mm ureteroscopes without lithotripsy and enhanced surgical techniques such as TIA or TIFA, with higher failure and conversion rates. There was no mentoring or hands on courses available in LBDE at that time. Furthermore, there was little or no organisational infrastructure that could support 'urgent/ semi-elective' cases in complex gallstone disease. The ability to perform these operations were often at the mercy of an emergency (CEPOD) list, with all the inherent challenges associated this this. The evolution of techniques and processes could only be realised by gaining real time operative experience and learning from patient outcomes. *Biliary Surgery 2.0* encompasses the overall strategy that has enabled a leading acute biliary service for complex gallstone disease at our institution (Fig. 7.20). LATEST is just a single element of *Biliary Surgery 2.0* and focuses on the technical aspects of the procedure in order to increase the transcystic exploration rate. In turn, this leads to better outcomes including reduced morbidity and shorter hospital admissions. As described in section "The impact of LBDE in a General Surgery department", the acute biliary pathway allows patients with acute biliary pathology admitted under our Emergency Surgery Unit (ESU) to be triaged into a dedicated 'biliary list'. The

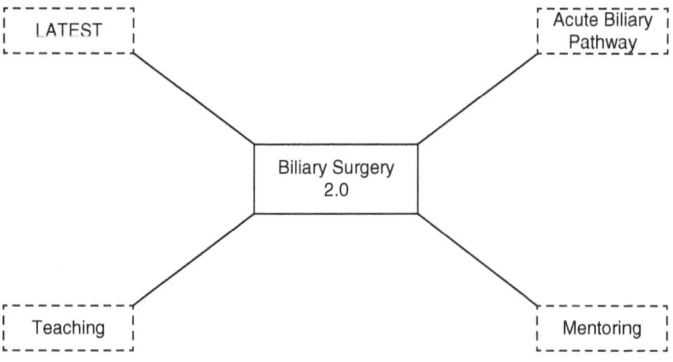

FIGURE 7.20 *Biliary Surgery 2.0*

biliary list consists of protected theatre sessions that effectively run like an emergency theatre and not scheduled with elective patients. The biliary list would require the availability of a radiographer and the C-arm to perform IOC which would be required in almost all patients. Furthermore, the equipment and staff required to perform lithotripsy (Holmium Laser Lithotripsy at our institution) would also be available including a laser-amenable theatre. Finally, teaching and mentoring are extremely important elements of *Biliary Surgery 2.0* and enable a 'shorter' learning curve, where the principles of LATEST becomes the main concentration. As described in section "Transcystic vs Transductal access", unpublished data from a surgeon at an institution outside of the UK who received our mentoring has achieved similar rates of transcystic exploration in their first 100 procedures compared to the last 100 from our series. Teaching and mentoring will be expanded further in Chap. 8.

References

1. NICE Clinical Guideline. Gallstones disease:Diagnosis and management. 2014.
2. Navaratne L, Martinez-Isla A. Transductal versus transcystic laparoscopic common bile duct exploration: an institutional review of over four hundred cases. Surg Endosc. 2020;35(1):437–48.
3. Zhu JG, Han W, Guo W, Su W, Bai ZG, Zhang ZT. Learning curve and outcome of laparoscopic transcystic common bile duct exploration for choledocholithiasis. Br J Surg. 2015;102(13):1691–7.
4. Liu W-S, Jiang Y, Zhang D, Shi L-Q, Sun D-L. Laparoscopic common bile duct exploration is a safe and effective strategy for elderly patients. Surg Innov [Internet]. 2018;25(5):465–9. Available from. https://doi.org/10.1177/1553350618785487.
5. Zhu H, Xu M, Shen H, Yang C, Li F, Li K, et al. A meta-analysis of single-stage versus two-stage management for concomitant gallstones and common bile duct stones. Clin Res Hepatol Gastroenterol. 2015;39(5):584–93.
6. Singh A, Kilambi R. Single-stage laparoscopic common bile duct exploration and cholecystectomy versus two-stage endoscopic

stone extraction followed by laparoscopic cholecystectomy for patients with gallbladder stones with common bile duct stones: systematic review and meta. Surg Endosc [Internet]. 2018;32(9):3763–76. Available from:. https://doi.org/10.1007/s00464-018-6170-8.

7. Prasson P, Bai X, Zhang Q, Liang T. One-stage laproendoscopic procedure versus two-stage procedure in the management for gallstone disease and biliary duct calculi: a systemic review and meta-analysis. Surg Endosc. 2016;30(8):3582–90.

8. Noble H, Tranter S, Chesworth T, Norton S, Thompson M. A randomized, clinical trial to compare endoscopic sphincterotomy and subsequent laparoscopic cholecystectomy with primary laparoscopic bile duct exploration during cholecystectomy in higher risk patients with choledocholithiasis. J Laparoendosc Adv Surg Tech [Internet]. 2009;19(6):713–20. Available from: http://www.liebertonline.com/doi/abs/10.1089/lap.2008.0428

9. Nagaraja V, Eslick G, Cox M. Systematic review and meta-analysis of minimally invasive techniques for the management of cholecysto-choledocholithiasis. J Hepatobiliary Pancreat Sci. 2014;21(12):896–901.

10. Dasari B, Tan CJ, Gurusamy KS, Martin DJ, Kirk G, Mckie L, et al. Surgical versus endoscopic treatment of bile duct stones (Review) SUMMARY OF FINDINGS FOR THE MAIN COMPARISON. Cochrane Database Syst Rev. 2013;12:CD003327.

11. Karvounis E, Griniatsos J, Arnold J, Atkin G, Marrtinez-Isla A. Why does laparoscopic common bile duct exploration fail? Int Surg. 2006;91(2):90–3.

12. Parra-Menbrives P, Martinez-Baena D, Lorente-Herce JM, Jimenez Mena GSM. Recurrencia de coledocolitiasis tras exploración laparoscópica de la vía biliar principal. Cir Esp. 2019;24 April.

13. Decker G, Borie F, Millat B, Berthou J, Deleuze ADF. One hundred laparoscopic choledochoyomies with primary closure of the common bile duct. Surg Endosc. 2003;17:12–8.

14. Dorman JP, Franklin MEGJ. Laparoscopic common bile duct exploration by choledochotomy. Surg Endosc. 1998;12:926–8.

15. Bansal V, Misra M, Garg P, Prabhu M. A prospective randomized trial comparing two-stage versus single-stage management of patients with gallstone disease and common bile duct stones. Surg Endosc. 2010;24(8):1986–9.

16. Bansal V, Misra M, Rajan K, Kilambi R, Kumar S, Krishna A, et al. Single-stage laparoscopic common bile duct exploration and cholecystectomy versus two-stage endoscopic stone extraction followed by laparoscopic cholecystectomy for patients with concomitant gallbladder stones and common bile duct stones: a randomized con. Surg Endosc. 2014;28(3):875–85.

17. Carroll BJ, Phillips E, Chandra MFM. Laparoscopic transcystic duct balloon dilatation of the sphincter of Oddi. Surg Endosc. 1993;7:514–7.

18. Rhodes M, Nathanson L, O'Rurke NF. Laparoscopic exploration of the common bile duct:lessons learned from 129 consecutive cases. Br J Surg. 1995;82:666–8.

19. Curet MJ, Pitcher DF, martin DT ZK. Laparoscopic antegrade sphincterotomy: a new technique for the management for complex choledocholithiasis. Ann Surg. 1995;221:149–55.

20. Gigot JF, Navez B, Etienne J, Cambier E, Jadoul GP, et al. A stratified intraoperative surgical strategy is mandatory during laparoscopic common bile duct exploration for common bile duct stones. Lessons and limits from an initial experience of 92 patients. Surg Endosc. 1997;11:722–8.

21. Neuhaus H, Hoffmann W, Zillinger C, Classen M. Laser lithotripsy of difficult bile duct stones under direct visual control. Gut. 1993;34(3):415–21.

22. Phillips EH, Roshenthal RJ, Carroll BJFM. Laparoscopic transcystic duct common bile duct exploration. Surg Endosc. 1994;8:1389–94.

23. Jones T, Al Musawi J, Navaratne L, Martinez-Isla A. Holmium laser lithotripsy improves the rate of successful transcystic laparoscopic common bile duct exploration. Langenbeck's Arch Surg. 2019;404(8):985–92.

24. Navarro-Sánchez A, Ashrafian H, Segura-Sampedro J, Martrinez-Isla A. LABEL procedure: laser-assisted bile duct exploration by Laparoendoscopy for choledocholithiasis: improving surgical outcomes and reducing technical failure. Surg Endosc. 2017;31(5):2103–8.

25. Martinez-Isla A, Martinez Cecilia D, Vilaça J, Navaratne LNSA. Laser-assisted bile duct exploration using laparoendoscopy LABEL technique, different scenarios and technical details. Epublication Websurgcom [Internet]. 2018;18(03) Available from: http://websurg.com/doi/vd01en5197

26. Martínez-Cecilia D, Navaratne L, Martínez Isla A. Biliary surgery 2.0. Cir Esp. 2020:2019–21.

27. Navaratne L, Al-Musawi J, Martinez Isla A. Comment on conventional surgical management of bile duct stones: a service model and outcomes of 1318 laparoscopic explorations no title. Ann Surg. 2021;

28. Ashby BS. Operative choledochoscopy in common bile duct surgery. Ann R Coll Surg Engl. 1985;67:279–83.

29. Lyu Y, Cheng Y, Li T, Cheng B, Jin X. Laparoscopic common bile duct exploration plus cholecystectomy versus endoscopic retrograde cholangiopancreatography plus laparoscopic cholecystectomy for cholecystocholedocholithiasis: a meta-analysis. Surg Endosc. 2019;33(10):3275–86.

30. Li ZQ, Sun JX, Li B, Dai XQ, Yu AX, Li ZF. Meta-analysis of single-stage versus two-staged management for concomitant gallstones abd common bile duct stones. J Minim Access Surg. 2019;

31. Gao YC, Chen J, Qin Q, Chen H, Wang W, Zhao J, et al. Efficacy and safety of laparoscopic bile duct exploration versus endoscopic sphincterotomy for concomitant gallstones and common bile duct stones. Med (United States). 2017;96(37)

32. Zhu J, Li G, Du P, Zhou X, Xiao W, Li Y. Laparoscopic common bile duct exploration versus intraoperative endoscopic retrograde cholangiopancreatography in patients with gallbladder and common bile duct stones: a meta-analysis. Surg Endosc. 2021;35(3):997–1005.

33. Liu J, Wang Y, Shu G, Lou C, Zhang J, Du Z. Laparoscopic versus endoscopic Management of Choledocholithiasis in patients undergoing laparoscopic cholecystectomy: a meta-analysis. J Laparoendosc Adv Surg Tech [Internet]. 2014;24(5):287–94. Available from: http://online.liebertpub.com/doi/abs/10.1089/lap.2013.0546

34. Reinders JSK, Gouma D, Ubbink DT, Van Ramshort B, Boerma D. Transcystic or transductal stone extraction during single stage treatment of choledochocystolithiasis: a systematic review. World J Surg. 2014;38:2403–11.

35. Pang L, Zhang Y, Wang Y, Kong J. Transcystic versus traditional laparoscopic common bile duct exploration: its advantages and a meta-analysis. Surg Endosc. 2018;32:4363–76.

36. Glomsaker T, Hoff G, Kvaloy T, Soreide KAJ. Patterns and predictive factors of complications after endoscopic retrograde cholangiopancreatopgraphy. Br J Surg. 2013;100:373–80.

37. Holdsworth RJ, Sadek SA, Ambikar SCA. Dynamics of bile flow through the human choledochal sphincter following exploration of the common bile duct. World J Surg. 1989;13:300–6.

38. De Roover D, Vanderveken MGY. Choledochotomy: primary closure versus T-tube. A prospective trial. Acta Chir Belg. 1989;89:320–4.
39. Paganini AM, Feliciotti F, Guerrieri M, Tamburini A, De Sanctis ACR, et al. Laparoscopic common bile duct exploration. J Laparoendosc Adv Surg Tech. 2001;11:391–400.
40. Isla A, Griniatsos J, Karvounis E, Arbuckle J. Advantages of laparoscopic stented choledochorrhaphy over T-tube placement. Br J Surg. 2004;91(7):862–6.
41. Treckmann P, Sauerland S, Frilling A, Paul A. Common bile duct stones-update 2006. In: Neugebauer E, Sauerland S, Fingerhut A, Millat B, Buess G, editors. EAES guidelines for endoscopic surgery twelve years evidence-based surgery in Europe. Heidelberg: Springer; 2006. p. 327–33.
42. Wills VL, Gibson K, Karihaloot C, Jorgensen J. Complications of biliary T-tubes after choledochotomy. Aust N Z J Surg. 2002;72:177–80.
43. Isla A, Griniatsos J, Wan A. A technique for safe placement of a biliary endoprosthesis after laparoscopic choledochotomy. J Laparoendosc Adv Surg Tech [Internet]. 2002;12(3):207–11. Available from: http://www.liebertpub.com/doi/10.1089/10926420260188128
44. Martínez Cecilia D, Valenti-Azcárate V, Qurashi K, Garcia-Agustí A, Marrtinez-isla A. Ventajas de la coledocorrafia laparoscópica sobre el stent. Experiencia tras seis años. Cir Esp. 2008;84(2):78–82.
45. Bernstein DE, Goldberg RI, Unger SW. Common bile duct obstruction following T-tube placement at laparoscopic cholecystectomy. Gastrointest Endosc. 1994;40:362–5.
46. Kacker LK, Mittal BR, Sikora SS, Ali W, Kapoor VK, Saxena R. Bile leak after T-tube removal a scintigraphic study. Hepato-Gastroenterology. 1995;42:975–8.
47. Mosimann F, Schneider R, Mir A, Gillet M. Erosion of the duodenum by a biliary T-tube: an unusual complication of liver transplantation. Transpl Proc. 1994;26:3550–1.
48. Ortega Lopez D, Ortiz Oshiro E, La Pena Gutierrez L, Martinez Sarmiento J, Sobrino del Riego JA, Alvarez Fernandez-Represa J. Scintigraphic detection of biliary fistula after removal of a T-tube. Br J Surg. 1995;82:82.
49. Lygidakis N. Choledochotomy for biliary lithiasis: T-tube drainage or primary closure. Effect on postoperative bacteremia and T-tube bile infection. Am J Surg. 1983;146:254–6.

50. DePaula AL, Hashiba K, Bafutto M, Machado C, Ferrari A, Machado M. Results of the routine use of a modified endoprosthesis to drain the common bile duct after laparoscopic choledochotomy. Surg Endosc. 1998;12:933–5.
51. Sheen-Chen S, Chou FF. Choledochotomy for biliary lithiasis: is routine T-tube drainage necessary? A prospective controlled trial. Acta Chir Scand. 1990;156:387–90.
52. Sheridan WG, Williams HO, Lewis MH. Morbidity and mortality of common bile duct exploration. Br J Surg. 1987;74:1095–9.
53. Abellán Morcillo I, Qurashi K, Martinez Isla A, Exploración laparoscópica de la vía biliar, lecciones aprendidas tras más de 200 casos. Cir Esp. 2014;92(5):341–44. https://doi.org/10.1016/j.ciresp.2013.02.010.
54. Banks PA, Bollen TL, Dervenis C, Gooszen HG, Johnson CD, Sarr MG, et al. Classification of acute pancreatitis--2012: revision of the Atlanta classification and definitions by international consensus. Gut. 2013 Jan;62(1):102–11.
55. Yin Z, Xu K, Sun J, Zhang J, Xiao Z, Wang J, Niu H, Zhao Q, Lin S, Li Y. Is the end for the T-tube drainage era in laparoscopic choledochotomy for common bile duct stones is coming? A systematic review and meta-analysys. Ann Surg. 2013;257:54–66.
56. Huihua C, Donglin S, Yuemin S, Bai J, Zhao HMY. Primary closure followinglaparoscopic common bile duct exploration combined with intraoperative cholangiography and choledochoscopy. World J Surg. 2012;36:164–70.
57. Wei Jie Z, Gui-Fang X, Guo-Zhong W, Jie-Ming L, Zhi-Tao D, Xiao-Dong M. Laparoscopic exploration of common bile duct with primary closure versus T tube drainage: a randomized clinical trial. J Surg Res. 2009;157(1):e1–5.
58. Koch M, Garden OJ, Padbury R, Rahbari NN, Adam R, Capussotti L, et al. Bile leakage after hepatobiliary and pancreatic surgery: a definition and grading of severity by the international study group of liver surgery. Surgery. 2011;149(5):680–8.
59. Parra-Membrives P, Martínez-Baena D, Lorente-Herce J, Martín-Balbuena R. Eficacia del sellante de fibrina-colágeno para reducir la incidencia de fístulas biliares tras la exploración laparoscópica de la vía biliar. Cirugía Española [Internet]. 2018;96(7):429–35. Available from: https://linkinghub.elsevier.com/retrieve/pii/S0009739X18301167
60. Martinez Isla A, Navaratne L, Quinones L, Martinez-Cecilia D. Carta al director: Eficacia del sellante de fibrina colageno para reducir la incidencia de fistulas biliares tras la exploracion laparosocpica de la via biliar. Cir Esp. 2019;97(2):119–24.

61. Navaratne L, Al-Musawi J, Acosta-Mérida A, Vilaça J, Martinez-Isla A. Trans-infundibular choledochoscopy: a method for accessing the common bile duct in complex cases. Langenbeck's Arch Surg. 2018;403(6):777–83.

62. Longland CJ. Choledochoscopy in choledocholithiasis. Br J Surg. 1973;60(8):626–8.

63. Rogers SJ, Cello JP, Horn JK, Siperstein AE, Schecter WP, Campbell AR, et al. Prospective randomized trial of LC+LCBDE vs ERCP/S+LC for common bile duct stone disease. Arch Surg. 2010;145(1):28–33.

64. Hongjun H, Yong J, Baoqiang W. Laparoscopic common bile duct exploration: choledochotomy versus transcystic approach? Surg Laparosc Endosc Percutan Tech. 2015;25(3):218–22.

65. Michalowski K, Bornmann PC, Krige JE, Gallagher PJ, Terblanche J. Laparoscopic subtotal cholecysetctomy in patients with complicated acute cholecystitisor fibrosis. Br J Surg. 1988;85:904–6.

66. Elsaher M, Gravante G, Thomas K, Sorge R, Al-Hamali S, Ebdewi H. Subtotal cholecystectomy for "difficult gallbladders" systematic review and meta analysis. JAMA Surg. 2015;150:159–68.

67. Shingu Y, Komatsu S, Norimizu S, Taguchi YS. Laparoscopic subtotal cholecystectomy for severe cholecystitis. Surg Endosc. 2016;30:526–31.

68. Hirajima S, Koh T, Sakai T, Imamura T, Kato S, Nishimura Y, Sogak NM, Oguro A, Nakagawa N. Utility of laparoscopic subtotal cholecystectomy with or without cystic duct ligation for severe cholecystitis. Am Surg. 2017;83:1209–13.

69. Chen D, Fei Z, Huang X, Wang X. Transcystic approach to laparosocpic common bile duct exploration. JSLS. 2014;

70. Senra F, Navaratne L, Acosta AMA. Laparoscopic management of type II Mirizzi syndrome. Surg Endosc [Internet]. 2020; Available from: https://doi.org/10.1007/s00464-019-07316-6

71. Williams E, Beckingham I, El Sayed G, et al. Updated guideline on the management of common bile duct stones (CBDS). Gut. 2017;66:765–82.

72. Ricci C, Pagano N, Taffurelli G, Pacilio C, Migliori M, Bazzoli F, et al. Comparison of efficacy and safety of 4 combinations of laparoscopic and intraoperative techniques for management of Gallstone Disease with Biliary Duct Calculi. JAMA Surg [Internet]. 2018:e181167. Available from: http://archsurg.jama-network.com/article.aspx?doi=10.1001/jamasurg.2018.1167

73. Navaratne L, Martinez IA. 10 years of laparoscopic bile duct exploration: a single tertiary institution experience. Am J Surg. 2019;

74. Cuschieri A, Lezoche E, Morino M, Croce E, Lacy A, Toouli J, et al. E.A.E.S. multicenter prospective randomized trial comparing two-stage vs single-stage management of patients with gallstone disease and ductal calculi. Surg Endosc. 1999;13(10):952–7.

75. Rhodes M, Sussman L, Cohen LLM. Randomised trial of laparoscopic exploration of common bile duct versus postoperative endoscopic retrograde cholangiography for common bile duct stones. Lancet. 1998;351:159–61.

76. Poh BR, Ho SPS, Sritharan M, Yeong CC, Swan MP, Devonshire DA, et al. Randomized clinical trial of intraoperative endoscopic retrograde cholangiopancreatography versus laparoscopic bile duct exploration in patients with choledocholithiasis. Br J Surg. 2016;103(9):1117–24.

77. Nathanson L, O'Rourke N, Martin I, Fielding G, Cowen A, Roberts R, et al. Postoperative ERCP versus laparoscopic choledochotomy for clearance of selected bile duct calculi: a randomized trial. Ann Surg. 2005;242(2):188–92.

78. Paganini AM, Guerrieri M, Sarnari J, De Sanctis A, D'Ambrosio G, Lezoche G, et al. Thirteen years' experience with laparoscopic transcystic common bile duct exploration for stones. Surg Endosc [Internet]. 2007;21(1):34–40. Available from: https://doi.org/10.1007/s00464-005-0286-3

79. Qandeel H, Zino S, Hanif Z, Nassar MKNA. Basket-in-catheter access for transcystic laparoscopic bile duct exploration: technique and results. Surg Endosc. 2016;30:1958–64.

80. Hajibandeh S, Hajibandeh S, Sarma DR, Balakrishnan S, Eltair M, Mankotia R, Budhoo MKY. Laparoscopic transcystic versus transductalcommon bile duct exploration:A systrematic review and meta-analysis. World J Surg 2019;Published.

81. Zhang WJ, Xu GF, Huang Q, Luo KL, Dong ZT, Li JM, Wu GZGW. Treatment of gallbladder stone with common bile duct stones in the laparoscopic era. BMC Surg. 2015;26(15):7.

82. Csendes A, Diaz JC, Burdiles P, Maluenda F, Nava O. Mirizzi syndrome and cholecystobiliary fistula: a unifying classification. Br J Surg. 1989;76(11):1139–43.

83. Lledó J, Barber S, Ibañez J, Torregrosa A, Lopez-Andujar R. Update on the diagnosis and treatment of Mirizzi syndrome in laparoscopic era: our experience in 7 years. Surg Laparosc Endosc Percutaneous Tech. 2014;24(6):495–501.

84. Payá-Llorente C, Vázquez-Tarragón A, Alberola-Soler A, Martínez-Pérez A, Martínez-López E, Santarrufina-Martínez S, et al. Mirizzi syndrome: a new insight provided by a novel classification. Ann Hepatobiliary Pancreatic Surg [Internet]. 2017;21(2):67–75.PMC5449366.
85. McSherry CK, Ferstenberg HVM. The Mirizzi syndrome:suggested classification and surgical therapy. Surg Gastroenterol. 1982;1:219–5.
86. Beltran MA, Csendes A, Cruces KS. The relationship of Mirizzi syndrome and cholecystoenteric fistula: validation of a modified classification. World J Surg. 2008;32(10):2237–43.
87. Beltrán MA. Mirizzi syndrome: history, current knowledge and proposal of a simplified classification. World J Gastroenterol. 2012;18(34):4639–50.
88. Shirah BH, Shirah HA, Albeladi KB. Mirizzi syndrome: necessity for safe approach in dealing with diagnostic and treatment challenges. Ann Hepato-Biliary-Pancreatic Surg. 2017;21(3):122.
89. Erben Y, Reid-Lombardo K, Que FG, Donohue JM, Farnell MB, Kendrick ML, et al. Diagnosis and treatment of Mirizzi syndrome: 23-year Mayo Clinic experience. J Am Coll Surg [Internet] 2011;213(1):114–119. Available from: https://doi.org/10.1016/j.jamcollsurg.2011.03.008
90. Kumar A, Senthil G, Prakash A, Behari A, Singh R, Kapoor V, et al. Mirizzi's syndrome: lessons learnt from 169 patients at a single center. Korean J Hepato-Biliary-Pancreatic Surg. 2016;20(1):17.
91. Kulkarni S, Hotta M, Sher L, Selby R, Parekh D, Buxbaum J, et al. Complicated gallstone disease: diagnosis and management of Mirizzi syndrome. Surg Endosc. 2017;31(5):2215–22.
92. Antoniou SA, Antoniou GA, Makridis C. Laparoscopic treatment of Mirizzi syndrome: a systematic review. Surg Endosc. 2010 Jan;24(1):33–9.
93. Lledó J, Barber S, Ibañez J, Torregrosa A, Lopez-Andujar R. Update on the diagnosis and treatment of Mirizzi syndrome in laparoscopic era: our experience in 7 years. Surg Laparosc Endosc Percutaneous Tech [Internet]. 2014;24(6):495–501. Available from: http://www.embase.com/search/results?subaction=viewrecord&from=export&id=L600770119%0Ahttp://sfx.library.uu.nl/utrecht?sid=EMBASE&issn=15344908&id=doi:&atitle=Update+on+the+diagnosis+and+treatment+of+Mirizzi+syndrome+in+laparoscopic+era%3A+Our+experience+

94. Cui Y, Liu Y, Li Z, Zhao E, Zhang H, Cui N. Appraisal of diagnosis and surgical approach for Mirizzi syndrome. ANZ J Surg. 2012;82(10):708–13.
95. Chowbey PK, Sharma A, Mann V, Khullar R, Baijal M, Vashistha A. The management of Mirizzi syndrome in the laparoscopic era. Surg Laparosc Endosc Percutan Tech. 2000;10(1):11–4.
96. Chuang S, Yeh M, Chang C. Laparoscopic transfistulous bile duct exploration for Mirizzi syndrome type II: a simplified standardized technique. Surg Endosc. 2016;30(12):5635–46.
97. Yuan H, Yuan T, Sun X, Zheng M. A minimally invasive strategy for Mirizzi syndrome type II. Surg Laparosc Endosc Percutan Tech. 2016;26(3):248–52.
98. Varban O, Assimos D, Passman C, Westcott C. Laparoscopic common bile duct exploration and holmium laser lithotripsy: a novel approach to the management of common bile duct stones. Surg Endosc. 2010;24(7):1759–64.
99. Schäfer M, Schneiter R, Krähenbühl L. Incidence and management of Mirizzi syndrome during laparoscopic cholecystectomy. Surg Endosc Other Interv Tech. 2003;17(8):1186–90.
100. Ireland A of S of GB and. Emergency General Surgery - The future: A Consensus Statement [Internet]. 2007. Available from: http://www.asgbi.org.uk/en/publications/consensus_statements.cfm
101. Anderson IMI. Emergency general surgery, Issues in professional practice.
102. AUGIS. Acute-Gallstones-Pathway-Final-Sept-2015.pdf [Internet]. Available from: http://www.augis.otg/wp-content/uploads/2014/05/Acute-gallstones-pathway-Final-Sept-2015.pdf
103. Hazra N, Gulliford M. Evaluating pancreatitis in primary care: a population-based cohort study Br J Gen Pract 2014;64(622):e295–310.
104. Sauerland S, Agresta F, Bergamaschi R, Borzellino G, Budzynski A, Champault G, et al. Laparoscopy for abdominal emergencies: evidence-based guidelines of the European Association for Endoscopic Surgery. Surg Endosc Other Interv Tech. 2006;20(1):14–29.
105. Working Party of the British Society of gastroenterology a of UGS of GB and I. UK guidelines for the management of acute pancreatitis. Gut 2005;1;54(suppl_3)):iii1–9.
106. Arbuckle J, Isla A. Acute Pancreatitis-Update 2006. In: Neugenbauer EAM, Sauerland S, Fingerhut A, Millat B, Buess

G, editors. EAES guidelines for endoscopic Sur- gery twelve years evidence-based surgery in Europe. Berlin: Springer; 2006. p. 377–86.

107. Navarro-Sánchez A, Ashrafian H, Laliotis A, Qurashi K, Martinez-Isla A. Single-stage laparoscopic management of acute gallstone pancreatitis: outcomes at different timings. Hepatobiliary Pancreat Dis Int. 2016;15(3):297–301.

108. Isla A, Griniatsos J, Rodway A. Single-stage definitive lap-aroscopic Management in Mild Acute Biliary Pancreatitis. J Laparoendosc Adv Surg Tech [Internet]. 2003;13(2):77–81. Available from: http://www.liebertonline.com/doi/abs/10.1089/109264203764654687

109. Mofiidi R, Madhavan KK, Garden OJ, Parks RW. An audit of the management of patients with acute pancreatitis against national standards of practice. Br J Surg 2007;94(7):844–88.

110. Creedon LR, Neophytou C, leeder PC AA. Are we meet-ing the British Society of Gastroenterology guidelines for cholecystectomy post-gallstones pancreatitis? ANZ J Surg 2016;86(12):1024–7.

111. El-Dhuwaib Y, Deakin M, david G, Durkin D, Corless D SJ. Definitive management of gallstones pancreatitis in England. Ann R Coll Surg Eng 2012;94(6):402–6.

112. AUGIS. SWORD. Available from: http://www.augis.org/sword/

113. NCEPOD. Acute pancreatitis:treat the cause [Internet]. 2016. Available from: https://www.ncepod.org.uk/2016ap.htlm

114. Monkhouse SJW, Court EL, Dash I CN. Two-week target for laparoscopic cholecystectomy following gallstones pancreatits is achievable and cost neutral. Br J Surg 2009;96(7):751–5.

115. Berger S, Taborda Vidarte CA, Woolard S, Morse B, Chawla S. Same-admission cholecystectomy compared with delayed cholecystectomy in acute gallstone pancreatitis: outcomes and predictors in a safety net hospital cohort. South Med J [Internet] 2020 Feb;113(2):87–92. Available from: https://doi.org/10.14423/SMJ.0000000000001067.

116. Murphy PB, Paskar D, Hilsden R, Koichopolos J, mele T. Western Ontario research collaborative on acute care Surgey:a means for providing cost-effective, quality care for gallstone pancre-atitis. World J Emerg Surg. 2017;Dec 28;12(1):20.

Chapter 8
Training in Laparoscopic Bile Duct Exploration (LBDE)

Lalin Navaratne, David Martinez Cecilia, and Alberto Martinez-Isla

Trends in the Utility of Laparoscopic Bile Duct Exploration (LBDE)

A nationwide assessment of trends in choledocholithiasis management in the United States from 1998 to 2013 found that the overall use of common bile duct (CBD) exploration (open and laparoscopic) decreased from 39.8% of admissions in 1998 to 8.5% in 2013 [1]. Specifically, laparoscopic bile duct exploration (LBDE) decreased from 9.2% to 3% within the same duration. The decreasing trend in LBDE has resulted in surgeons being less experienced in performing this procedure. When it is undertaken, it is often at the expense of longer operative times and more complications [2]. Another study from the United States evaluated the

L. Navaratne (✉) · A. Martinez-Isla
Northwick Park and St Mark's Hospitals, London North West University Healthcare NHS Trust, London, UK
e-mail: lalin.navaratne@doctors.org.uk; a.isla@imperial.ac.uk

D. Martinez Cecilia
Hospital Universitario de Toledo, Toledo, Spain

© The Author(s), under exclusive license to Springer Nature Switzerland AG 2022
A. Martinez-Isla, L. Navaratne (eds.), *Laparoscopic Common Bile Duct Exploration*, In Clinical Practice,
https://doi.org/10.1007/978-3-030-93203-9_8

impact of declining CBD exploration from 2000 to 2018 on surgical training in bile duct procedures [3]. Despite an increase in the number of laparoscopic cholecystectomies performed per general surgery resident (84 to 117; 39%), the mean number of cases for open and laparoscopic CBD exploration per general surgery resident decreased (2.7 to 0.7; 74% and 0.9 to 0.7; 22% respectively). Therefore, general surgery residents in the United States, on average, perform less than one LBDE during their entire training, which has also been confirmed by other authors [4]. Consequently, it is not surprising that 86% of general surgeons in the United States chose pre-operative endoscopic retrograde cholangio-pancreatography (ERCP) as the management of choice for pre-operatively known choledocholithiasis in a web-based survey [5]. The situation in the United Kingdom is likely to be similar. In order to promote single-stage management (laparoscopic cholecystectomy + LBDE) of choledocholi-thiasis and increase its widespread adoption, a comprehen-sive training program together with mentoring is needed. Training in LBDE should be available to consultants and senior specialist registrars (SpR) in General Surgery and can be delivered during surgical training as well as dedicated LBDE training courses. A reliable and reproducible LBDE training model should be used to facilitate learning and enable translation of acquired skills into clinical practice. The use of a LBDE curriculum has been shown to improve the ability of surgeons to perform both transductal and tran-scystic exploration on a procedural simulator and increase the institutional utilisation of LBDE [6, 7].

Simulation Training in LBDE: The Porcine Aorto-Renal Artery (PARA) Model

In the UK, NICE guidelines recommend LBDE at the time of laparoscopic cholecystectomy for the management of cho-ledocholithiasis with concomitant gallstones, provided that the necessary expertise are available [8]. It has been discussed at great length throughout this book that LBDE should preferably be performed via the transcystic route. If expertise in LBDE is not available, then patients should be offered preoperative ERCP followed by laparoscopic cholecystectomy. An important factor for skill acquisition in LBDE, besides the theoretical knowledge, is the availability of a high fidelity, reliable and reproducible model for surgeons to undertake simulation training. Laparoscopic training boxes such as the Fundamentals of Laparoscopic Surgery (FLS) trainer box (VTI Medical, Waltham, Massachusetts, USA) can be complemented with a realistic, readily available model of the biliary tree for simulation training in LBDE.

Early models in LBDE were made from available medical devices such as urinary catheters and latex tubes; however, these models lacked realistic tissue-handling experience (face validity) [9, 10]. In 2014, we described a new model for training in LBDE using the porcine aorta [11]. The diameter and consistency of the porcine aorta resembles that of the human bile duct, making it ideal for training in transductal LBDE and flexible choledochoscopy. This model was successfully implemented within the Pan-London General Surgical Skills Training Programme and received good trainee feedback. Since then, increasing rates of transcystic LBDE called for a model specifically designed for training in transcystic techniques. The Porcine Aorto-Renal Artery (PARA) model is an evolution of the previous model enabling simulation training in both transcystic and transductal LBDE [12]. The unprepared specimen is obtained frozen and includes the whole porcine aorto-renal block (from ~60 kg pigs) at a cost of £18.50. For the preparation of the model, the peri-renal and peri-aortic fat is removed (Fig. 8.1), and the specimen is placed on a cork board. The left kidney with its renal artery is rotated 90° anti-clockwise to simulate the liver and common hepatic duct respectively (Fig. 8.2a). The supra-renal aorta is ligated at the level of the renal arteries (Fig. 8.2b*) and the distal infra-renal aorta is partially ligated to simulate the papilla. Finally, the right renal artery (at the level of the hilum) is elevated 40 mm to represent the anatomical

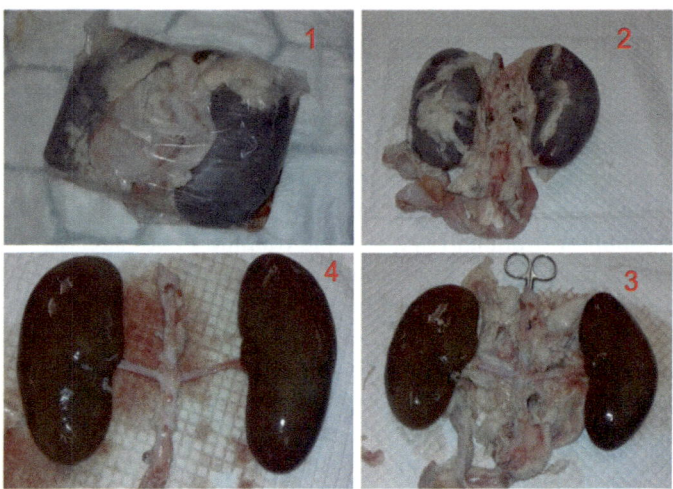

FIGURE 8.1 Aorto-renal block

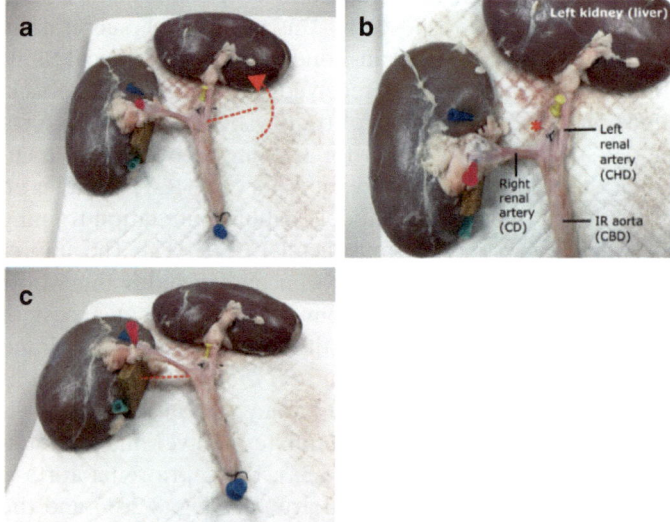

FIGURE 8.2 Rotation of the left kidney Will result in the left renal artery simulating the common hepatic duct

configuration of the cystic and common ducts (Fig. 8.2c). Peppercorns or chalk can be used to simulate CBD stones. Chalk was chosen as it simulates stones with high calcium content and provides realistic training in lithotripsy techniques.

Modular Training in Laparoscopic Bile Duct Exploration (LBDE)

The concept of modular training can be used to structure training. In modular training, a complex procedure is broken down into smaller steps ('modules') of mixed complexity, and mastering of the individual steps should result in the acquisition of skills required to achieve competency in the procedure. For training in LBDE, we use a modified version of a curriculum proposed by Teitelbaum et al. [6]. The procedure has been modularised into 14 steps which is summarised in Table 8.1 and Figs. 8.3, 8.4, 8.5, 8.6, 8.7, 8.8, 8.9, 8.10, 8.11, 8.12 and 8.13. The complete technical description of each step, explained fully elsewhere in this book, can be found in the right-hand column of Table 8.1. Table 8.2 summarises how the steps of the procedure are translated into practice using the PARA training model with a focus on common pitfalls and tips for trainees.

Gaining Competency in LBDE

Competency in LBDE can be achieved in three phases. Firstly, surgeons must understand the theoretical knowledge of LBDE: indications, rationale and evidence-base, equipment and devices, and technique. This book provides all the theoretical knowledge required to undertake LBDE. Much of the content of this book has also been delivered online in a series of pre-recorded [13, 14] and live ('*One-Stage Cholecystectomy and Laparoscopic Bile Duct Exploration Pathway Program*', Johnson & Johnson Institute) webinars.

TABLE 8.1 Training in LBDE: 14 steps

Step	Operative stage	Technical description
1	Placement of the cholangiogram needle (or a Belluci style 30° ENT disposable suction tube) through the abdominal wall aligned with the axis of the cystic duct	Section "Intra-operative cholangiogram (IOC)" in Chap. 4
2	Opening the cystic duct	Section "Intra-operative cholangiogram (IOC)" in Chap. 4
3	Cannulation of the cystic duct with a guidewire	Section "Intra-operative cholangiogram (IOC)" in Chap. 4
4	Cystic duct dilatation with a 12F access sheath	Section "Choledochoscopy" in Chap. 4 Section "Scenario 1: Both the cystic duct and CBD are not dilated" in Chap. 6
5	Transcystic (3 mm) choledochoscopy with distal and proximal views	Section "Scenario 1: Both the cystic duct and CBD are not dilated" in Chap. 6
6	Transcystic standard retrieval techniques: Capturing a stone using a Dormia basket	Section "Scenario 1: Both the cystic duct and CBD are not dilated" in Chap. 6
7	Transcystic standard retrieval techniques: Extraction of the captured stone	Section "Scenario 1: Both the cystic duct and CBD are not dilated" in Chap. 6
8	Cystic duct ligation	Section "Closure after the transcystic approach" in Chap. 6

TABLE 8.1 (continued)

Step	Operative stage	Technical description
9	Performing a choledochotomy	Section "Scenario 3: The cystic duct is not dilated but the CBD is dilated" in Chap. 6
10	Placement of a 5 mm port perpendicular to the choledochotomy	Section "Scenario 3: The cystic duct is not dilated but the CBD is dilated" in Chap. 6
11	Transductal choledochoscopy with distal and proximal views	Section "Scenario 3: The cystic duct is not dilated but the CBD is dilated" in Chap. 6
12	Transductal stone extraction using standard retrieval techniques	Section "Scenario 3: The cystic duct is not dilated but the CBD is dilated" in Chap. 6
13	Closure of choledochotomy	Section "Closure after accessing the bile duct" in Chap. 6
14	Lithotripsy-assisted bile duct exploration by Laparoendoscopy (LABEL)	Sections "Laser lithotripsy" and "Electrohydraulic lithotripsy (EHL)" in Chap. 4 Section "Surgical technique for LABEL" in Chap. 5

Secondly, surgeons will gain hands-on experience of LBDE using a simulation training model (e.g., PARA model). There are many courses available in LBDE and the first '*One-Stage Cholecystectomy and Laparoscopic Bile Duct Exploration Pathway Program*', by Johnson & Johnson Institute (AMI and LN were faculty) was completed in London in 2021. An outline of the program is summarised in Fig. 8.14. The second

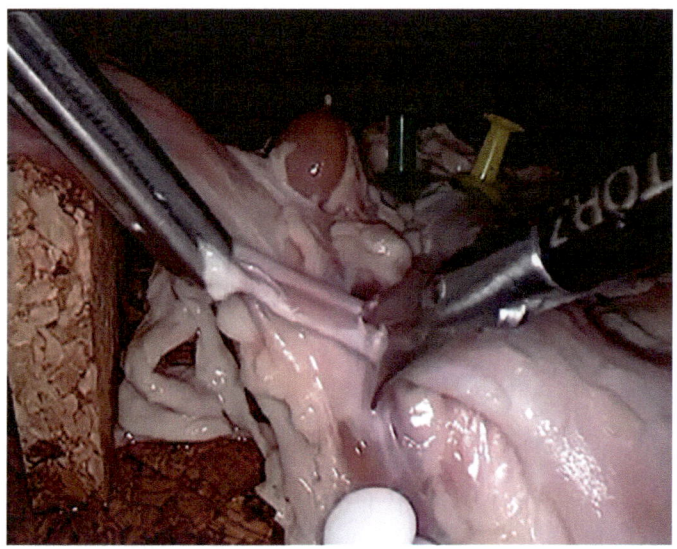

FIGURE 8.3 Opening the cystic duct

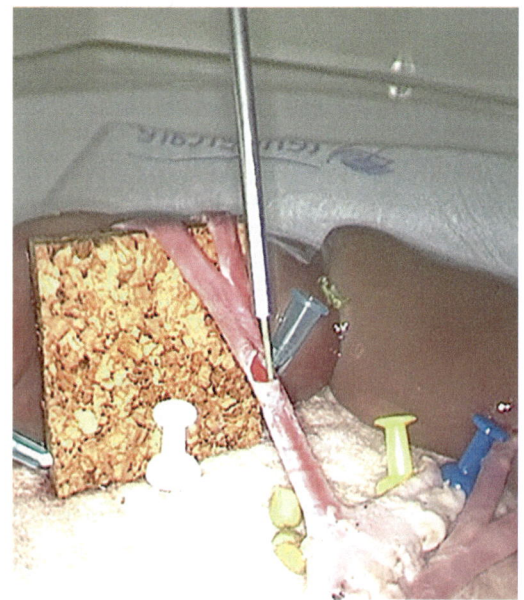

FIGURE 8.4 Cannulation of the cystic duct with a guidewire

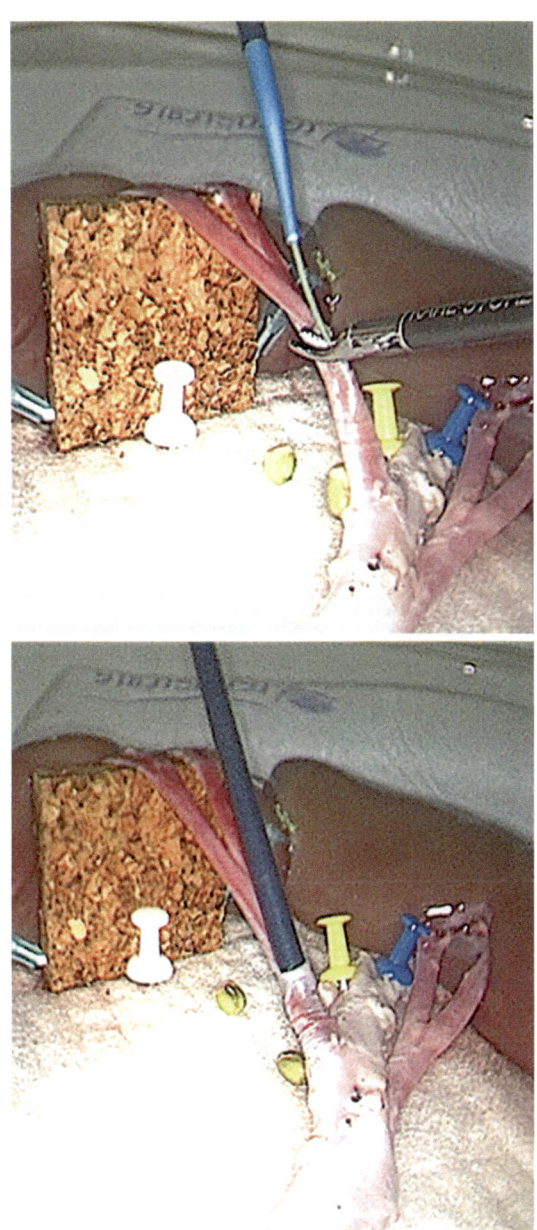

Figure 8.5 Cystic duct dilatation with a 12F access sheath

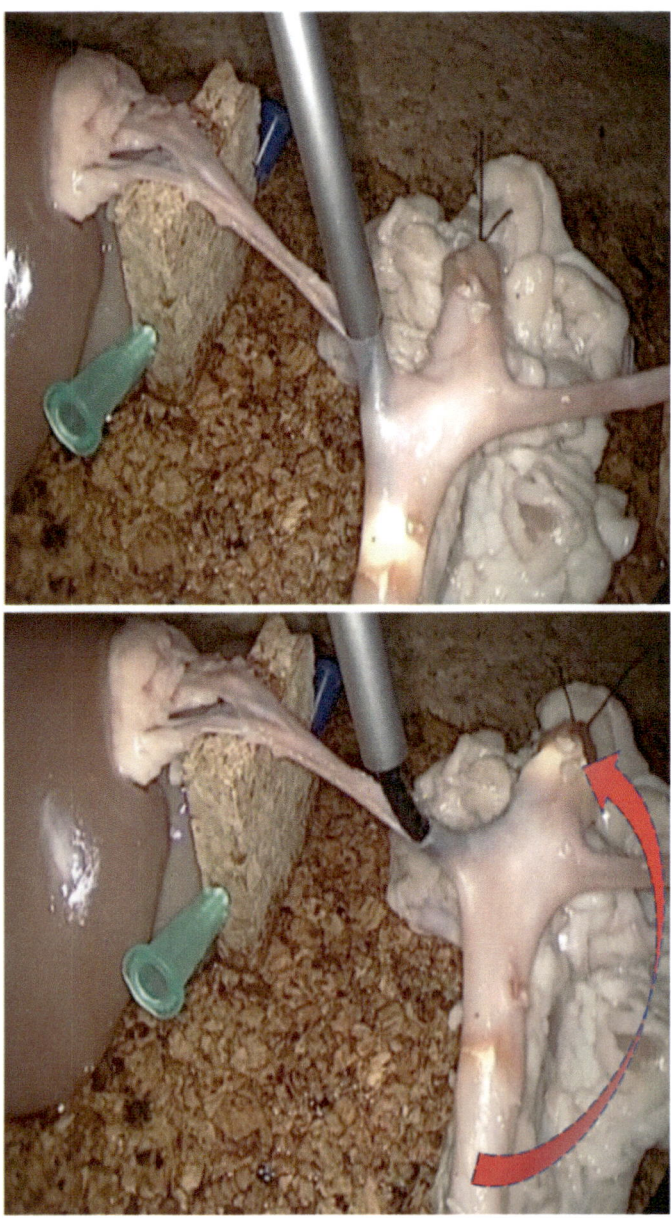

FIGURE 8.6 Transcystic (3 mm) choledochoscopy with distal and proximal views

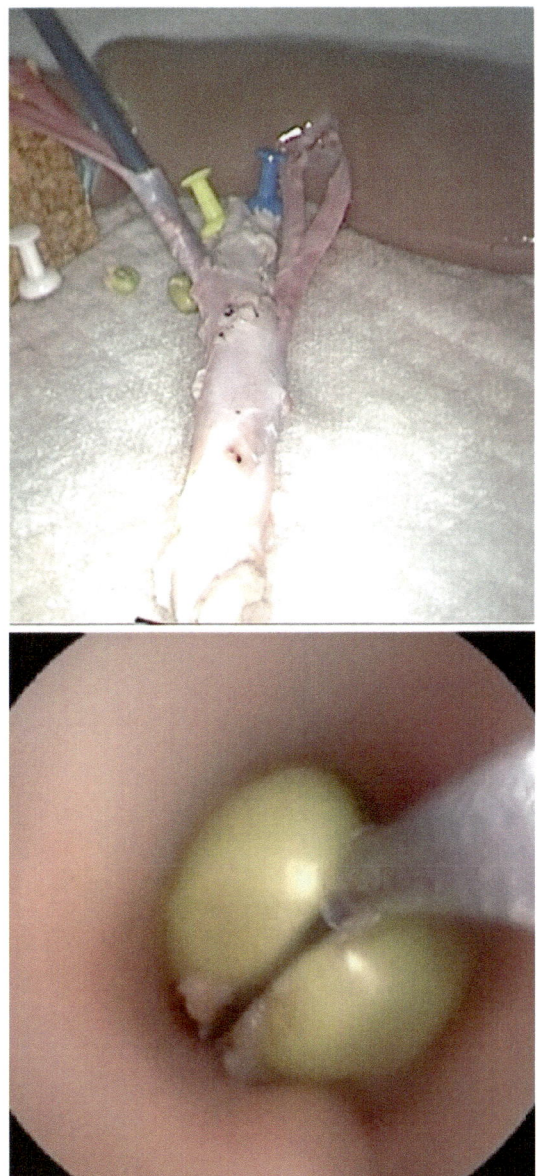

FIGURE 8.7 Transcystic standard retrieval techniques: capturing a stone using a Dormia basket

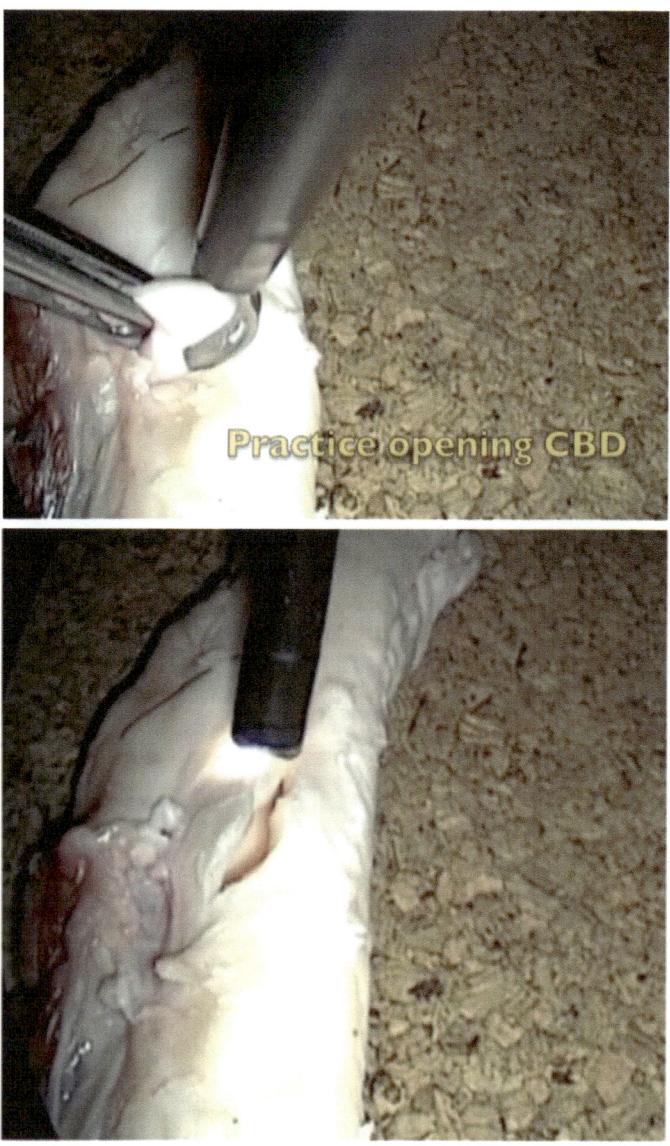

FIGURE 8.8 Performing a choledochotomy

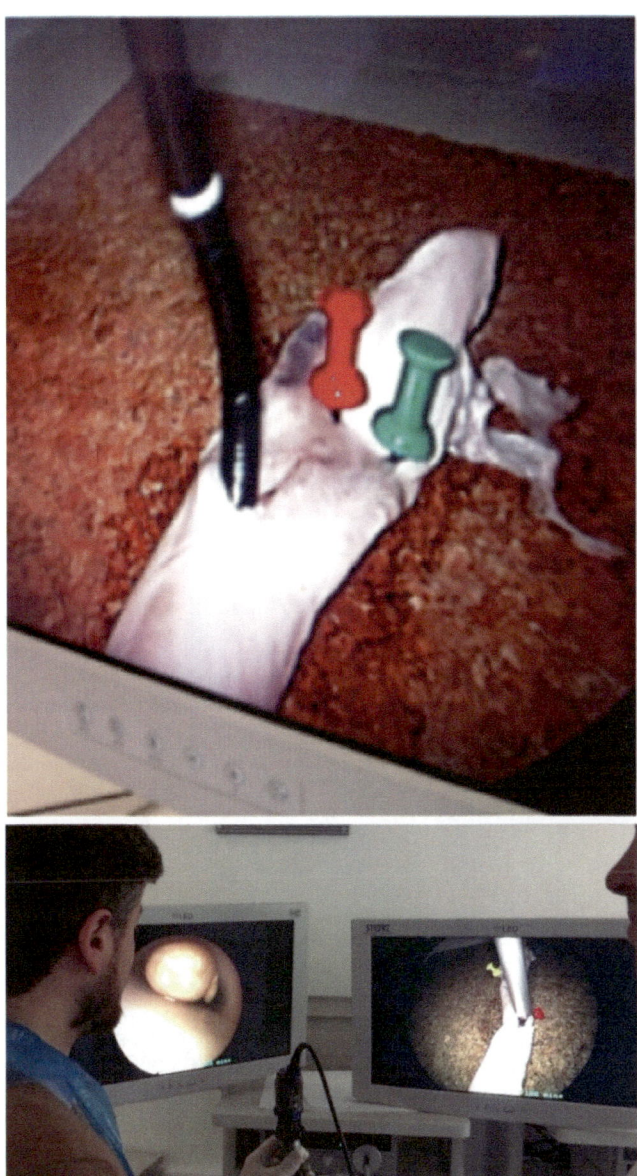

Figure 8.9 Transductal choledochoscopy with distal and proximal views

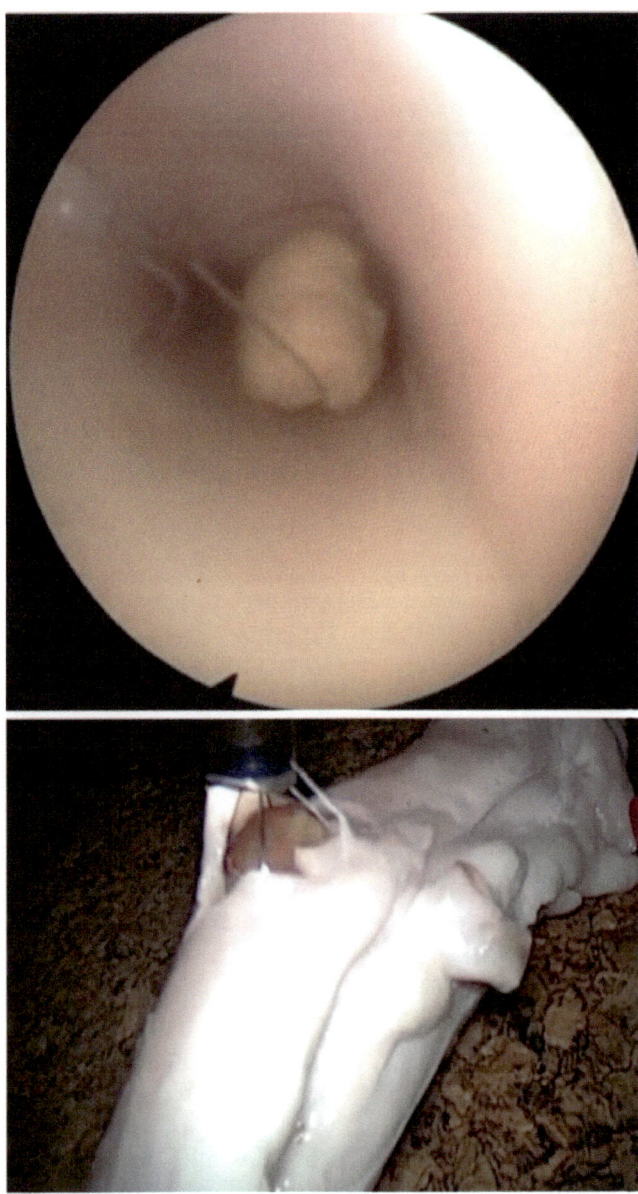

FIGURE 8.10 Transductal stone extraction using standard retrieval techniques

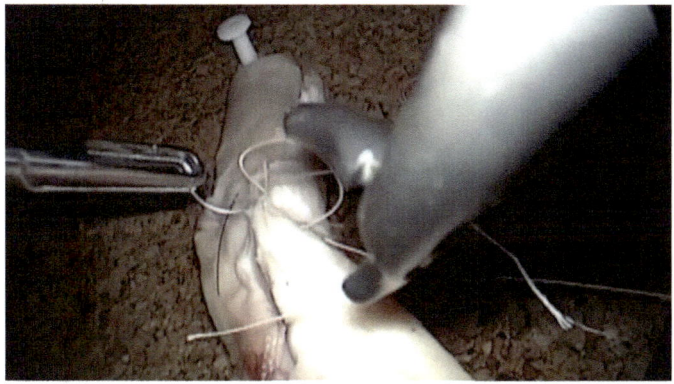

FIGURE 8.11 Closure choledochotomy

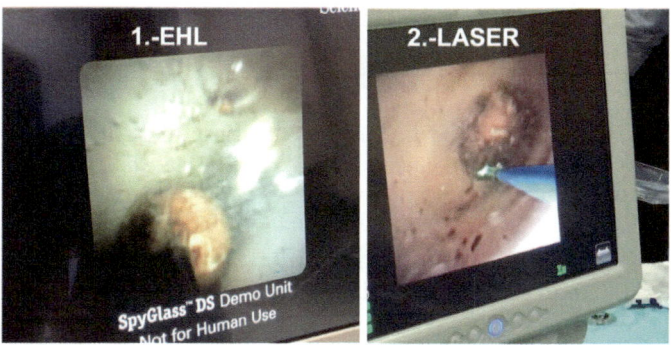

FIGURE 8.12 Lithotripsy-Assisted Bile duct Exploration by Laparoendoscopy (LABEL) with pepper corns simulating stones. Left, electrohydraulic lithotripsy (EHL). Right, holmium laser lithotripsy (HLL)

part of this programme consisted of a hands-on (face-to-face) course using the PARA model. We recommend following the modular training program as outlined in section "Modular training in Laparoscopic Bile Duct Exploration (LBDE)". Thirdly, and finally, surgeons should undertake procedural training in live patients. This will encompass supervised training and mentoring. For specialty registrars (residents) or post-Certificate of Completion of Training (post-CCT)

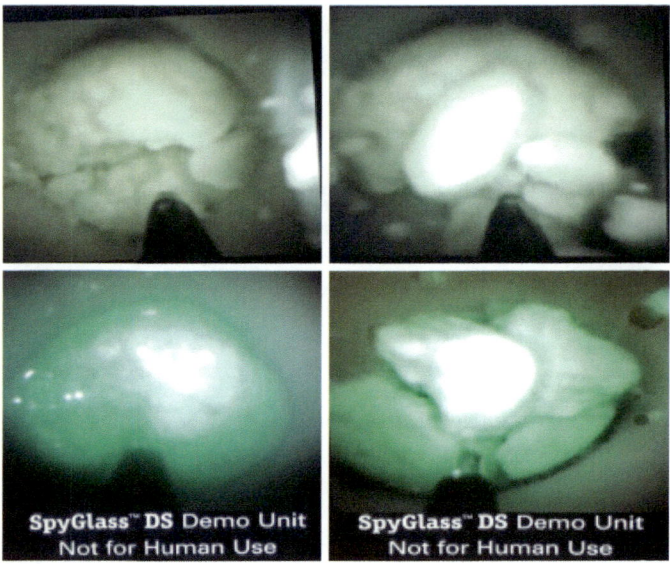

FIGURE 8.13 Simulation training in Lithotripsy-Assisted Bile duct Exploration by Laparoendoscopy (LABEL) using white (top) and green (bottom) chalk

fellows, rotating to institutions with an established LBDE practice will provide immediate exposure. Assisting in LBDE followed by supervised 'modular' training (see section "Modular training in Laparoscopic Bile Duct Exploration (LBDE)") should be the aim of the trainee. For others, a period of mentoring will enable safe practice and a quicker learning curve. Mentoring will involve the mentee visiting the mentor, and vice versa, to observe live surgery. Traditionally, this has been carried out in person, but emerging technologies such as Rods & Cones (a platform for audio and visual communication) enables 'virtual' mentoring anywhere in the world [15]. These platforms can provide experts in LBDE on-demand access to the operating theatre of the mentee (one-to-one) to provide advice and guidance in real-time. Similarly, the mentor can also live stream operations to an audience (one-to-many) providing mentorship to multiple

TABLE 8.2 Modular training in LBDE

Step	Operative stage	Learning points
1	Access through the abdominal wall: TC	Access through the abdominal wall is achieved using a cholangiogram needle or a Belluci style 30° ENT disposable suction tube. Trainees should focus on aligning the needle/suction tube to the axis of the cystic duct (which has been retracted through the abdominal wall using an Endoloop® and Endo close™ as previously described—see Chap. 4, section "Cholecystectomy") as this will determine the direction of the access sheath for the transcystic approach.
2	Opening the CD	The cystic duct is then opened with scissors (Fig. 8.3). Trainees should take care not to completely transect the cystic duct which is easily done if it is very thin.
3	CD guidewire cannulation	A guidewire is passed through the cholangiogram needle or ENT suction tube and the cystic duct is cannulated (Fig. 8.4). Trainees should practice co-ordinating the movement of the guidewire through the cholangiogram needle or ENT suction tube using one hand and the direction of the cholangiogram needle or ENT suction tube with the other hand. The model will allow trainees to practice performing an IOC. A 5F cholangiogram catheter (Tables 4.1–4.7) can be passed over the guidewire to lie in the CBD (with subsequent removal of the guidewire) in preparation for an IOC.

(continued)

TABLE 8.2 (continued)

Step	Operative stage	Learning points
4	CD dilatation	If a cholangiogram has been simulated, the guidewire will need to be re-introduced into the CBD by passing it through the cholangiogram catheter. Training in transcystic exploration is achieved by introducing the 12F access sheath (Tables 4.1–4.6) over the guidewire to gently dilate the cystic duct (Fig. 8.5). The 12F access sheath permits a 3 mm choledochoscope and therefore the cystic duct will need to be dilated to 4 mm (the 12F access sheath has an external diameter of 4 mm). This should be done gently and gradually and trainees should practice this step without causing complete transection of the cystic duct due to excessive traction.
5	TC choledochoscopy	Using the access sheath, a 3 mm choledochoscope is inserted into the CBD via the cystic duct (Fig. 8.6). Trainees should practice navigating the choledochoscope without directly grasping the shaft with a laparoscopic instrument, which will result in damaging the scope. Trainees should practice the 'windscreen wiper' manoeuvre to enable proximal choledochoscopy of the intra-hepatic ducts (Fig. 8.6 right).

TABLE 8.2 (continued)

Step	Operative stage	Learning points
6	TC stone capture	Simulated stones are be captured using a Dormia basket (Fig. 8.7). There are many varieties of baskets made by different manufacturers and trainees should become familiar with those likely to be used at their institution. Trainees should practice controlling the tip of the choledochoscope whilst introducing the basket through the working channel of the choledochoscope. A co-ordinated effort with the assistant controlling the opening and closing of the basket is required and should be practiced to ensure efficient stone capture.
7	TC stone extraction	The feasibility to extract captured stones through the cystic duct must be assessed. Extracting a large stone through a thinner cystic duct could result in impaction of the basket-stone complex (see Chap. 6, section "Scenario 3: The cystic duct is not dilated but the CBD is dilated"). The awareness of making this decision should be instilled in trainees. If the stone is deemed extractable by standard retrieval techniques, a co-ordinated extraction of the basket-stone complex along with the choledochoscope should be practiced in order to remove the stone. For larger stones, the LABEL technique will be required (see step 14).
8	CD ligation	Trainees should practice ligating the cystic duct with clips, an Endoloop® and suture ligation.

(continued)

TABLE 8.2 (continued)

Step	Operative stage	Learning points
9	Choledochotomy	Following training in steps 1–8 (transcystic LBDE), the same model can be used for training in transductal LBDE. The porcine aorta has great likeness to the human CBD and offers high fidelity training in tissue handing which cannot be provided by plastic models. A choledochotomy provides transductal access and can be performed using scissors (Fig. 8.8) or a Berci knife®. We recommend performing a longitudinal (vertical) choledochotomy but a horizontal incision can also be practiced.
10	Access through the abdominal wall: TD	Once a choledochotomy has been performed, a 3 or 5 mm choledochoscope can be used as the incision will be 5 mm or more. If a 5 mm port is utilised for insertion of the choledochoscope, it should be inserted through the abdominal wall so that it approaches the CBD at a 90° (perpendicular) angle (Fig. 8.9). The same principle applies if the 12F access sheath is used for 3 mm choledochoscopy.
11	TD choledochoscopy	Distal and proximal choledochoscopy should be practiced via the choledochotomy. Trainees should focus on manoeuvring the choledochoscope without directly grasping the shaft with forceps.
12	TD stone extraction	As with steps 6 and 7, trainees should practice the capture and extraction of stones through the choledochotomy using a Dormia basket (Fig. 8.10).

TABLE 8.2 (continued)

Step	Operative stage	Learning points
13	Closure of choledochotomy	Closure of choledochotomy will require competency in advanced laparoscopic suturing and the PARA model will provide trainees with high fidelity simulation. Trainees should practice primary closure with both interrupted and continuous suturing (Fig. 8.11). Trainees can also practice closure of choledochotomy over a T-tube and primary closure with a transcystic drain.
14	LABEL	The PARA model can be turned into a 'wet' model for training in lithotripsy (LABEL). Irrigation of saline from the choledochoscope is required for both holmium laser lithotripsy (HLL) and electrohydraulic lithotripsy (EHL). Figure 8.12 Demonstrates EHL (left) and HLL (right) to fragment peppercorns. Some CBD stones have very high calcium content (best appreciated on pre-operative imaging with CT), and this can be simulated by substituting pepper corns for chalk (Fig. 8.13). Trainees should familiarise themselves with the various equipment and devices needed to perform LABEL (see Chap. 4, sections "Laser lithotripsy" and "Electrohydraulic lithotripsy (EHL)") including all the safety aspects involved (especially with laser). If simulation is undertaken with laser, ensure all the appropriate precautions (e.g., goggles, room safety etc) are taken prior to starting the training.

TC transcystic, *CD* cystic duct, *IOC* intra-operative cholangiogram, *CBD* common bile duct, *TD* transductal, *LABEL* Lithotripsy-Assisted Bile duct Exploration by Laparoendoscopy

Johnson&Johnson

INSTITUTE

Virtual Program

Virtual Session 1: Background & Justification for Single Stage Approach

- History of bile duct exploration

- Advantages of single stage treatment over the traditional pre-operative ERCP + laparoscopic cholecystectomy for management of CBD stones

Virtual Session 2: Clinical Use of Lithotripsy & Energy

- LABEL: Laparoscopic Bile Duct Exploration by Laparoendoscopy: Principles and Technique

- Pre-LABEL: Factors predicting the use of lithotripsy during LBDE

- Clinical Cases (Interactive)

Virtual Session 2: Laser Lithotripsy: Principles and Safety

- Delivered by Dr Ismail Badr
- Introduction to Holmium YAG Laser
- General principal and safety of laser

Virtual Session 4: Introduction to Surgical Techniques

- Trascystic bile duct exploration
- Transductal bile duct exploration
    - Primary closure
    - Closure over T tube
    - Closure over anterograde stent
    - Closure and transcystic drain
- Different scenarios that can be found in LBDE
- Advance and instruction for the practical session

FIGURE 8.14 One-Stage Cholecystectomy and Laparoscopic Bile Duct Exploration Pathway Program. Johnson & Johnson Institute

surgeons at the same time. The devices are designed to be worn within the sterile environment of an operating theatre, are lightweight and hands free (Fig. 8.15). The one-to-many function of this technology can facilitate broadcasting of LBDE from an expert surgeon to mentees and would be the

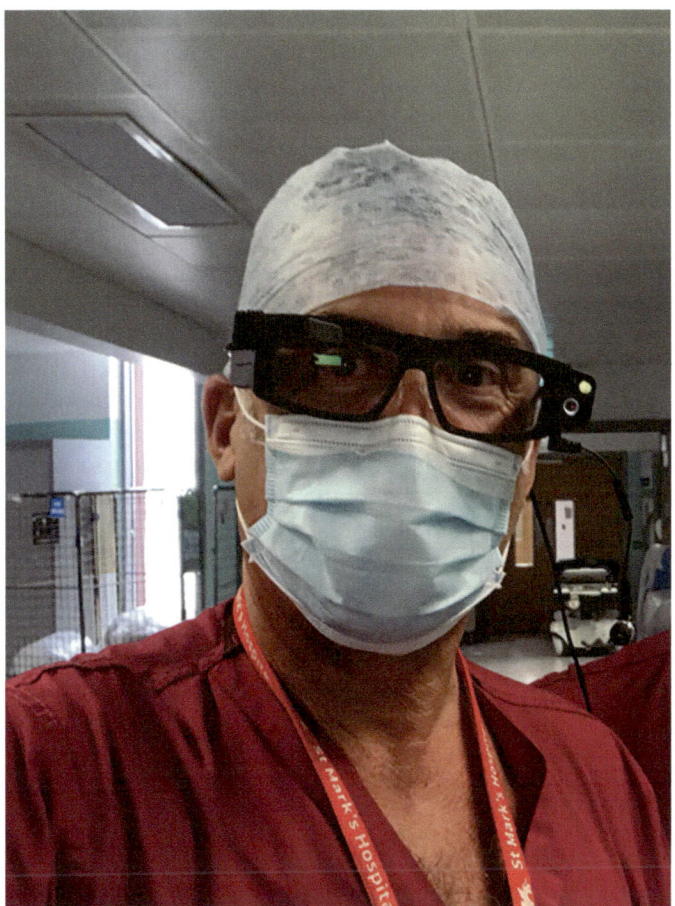

FIGURE 8.15 'Rods & Cones glasses'

ideal start to the third phase (following theoretical learning and hands-on simulation training). Other platforms such as 'Proximie' can also facilitate training and mentoring in LBDE. Proximie is a technology platform that allows surgeons to virtually 'scrub in' to any operating theatre from anywhere in the world [16]. This platform can empower experts in LBDE to share their skills in real-time, thereby standardising technique (such as the LATEST principles), reducing variation in care and improving patient outcomes. Used in reverse, the mentor can be present in the mentee's operating theatre and the virtual interaction afforded by this technology means that the mentor can physically guide the mentee in real-time. Finally, the Surgical Process Institute (SPI) is a platform from Johnson & Johnson that was developed to support surgeons and surgical teams through digitalised workflows, establishing optimum standards and promote continuous practical leaning [17]. The intuitively operable and modular platform allows for various processes (workflows) in the surgical theatre to be developed, digitized, and implemented together. All procedural steps are illustrated chronologically and documented, including any necessary deviations that may be required during the course of the operation. With our collaboration, the various steps of the LBDE procedure (modular training) have been entered onto this platform as the *surgeon's workflow* (Fig. 8.16). This can act as a 'digital' guidebook for surgeons who are beginning their independent practice. LBDE is a highly technical procedure that relies on various medical devices and equipment. The long list of devices and consumables can be intimidating to the novice surgeon and the nursing (scrub) staff. SPI allows the creation of digitalised workflows, including checklists of

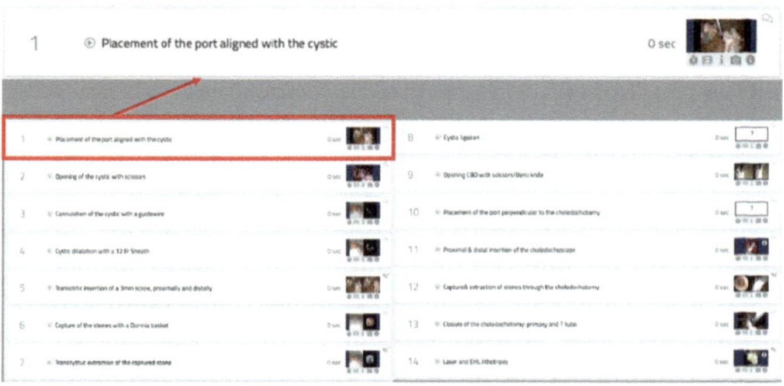

FIGURE 8.16 Surgical Process Institute (SPI): Modular training for LBDE using the PARA model

the equipment required, which can be tailored to the surgeon and appear on the *nurse's workflow*. The recent advances in digital health and mentoring platforms will facilitate wider uptake of single-stage management of choledocholithiasis and future work should focus on further developing educational platforms for training in LBDE.

References

1. Wanding MW, Hungness ES, Pavey ES, Stulberg JJ, Sschwab B, Yang AD, Shapiro MB, Billimoria KY, Ko CY, Nathens A. Nationwide assessment of trends in choledocholithiasis Management in the United States from 1998 to 2013. JAMA Surg. 2016;151(12):1125–30.
2. Herrero A, Phillipe C, Guillon F, Millat B, Borie F. Does the surgeon's experience influence the outcome of laparoscopic treatment of common bile duct stones? Surg Endosc. 2013;27:176–80.
3. Warner R, Coleman K, Musgrove K, Bardes J, Borgstrom D, Grabo D. A review of general surgery resident experience in common bile duct exploration in the ERCP era. Am J Surg [Internet] 2020;(xxxx). Available from: https://doi.org/10.1016/j.amjsurg.2020.02.032.
4. Helling TS, Khandelwal A. The challenges of resident training in complex hepatic, pancreatic, and biliary procedures. J Gastrointest Surg [Internet] 2008;12(1):153–158. Available from: https://doi.org/10.1007/s11605-007-0378-6.
5. Baucom RB, Feurer ID, Shelton JS, Kummerow K, Holzman MD, Poulose B. Surgeons, ERCP, and laparoscopic common bile duct exploration: do we need a standard approach for common bile duct stones? Surg Endosc. 2016;30(2):414–23.
6. Teitelbaum E, Soper N, Santos B, Rooney D, Patel P, Nagle A, et al. A simulator-based resident curriculum for laparoscopic common bile duct exploration. Surg (United States). 2014;156(4):880–93.
7. Schwab B, Teitelbaum E, Barsuk J, Soper N, Hungness E. Single-stage laparoscopic management of choledocholithiasis: an analysis after implementation of a mastery learning resident curriculum. Surg (United States). 2018;163(3):503–8.
8. NICE Clinical Guideline. Gallstones disease:Diagnosis and management. 2014.

9. Synder M, Hungness E, Santos B, Rosser J, Dunking B, Teitelbaum E. A Socially Distanced Approach to Surgical Education: A Hybrid Web and Simulator-Based Course for Laparoscopic Common Bile Duct Exploration [Internet]. Northwestern Medicine. Feinberg School of Medicine. Available from: https://www.surgery.northwestern.edu/docs/edelstone-bendix-research-poster/2021posters/snyder-2021.pdf

10. Perissat J, Collet D, Belliard R, Desplantez J. Laparoscopic cholecystectomy: the state of the art. A report on 700 consecutive cases. World J Surg. 1992;16:1074–82.

11. Navarro-sanchez A, Von-Roon A, Thomas R, Marchington S, Isla A. A new teaching model for laparoscopic common bile duct exploration: use of porcine aorta. Cirugía Española (English Ed [Internet]) 2014;92(10):692–693. Available from: https://doi.org/10.1016/j.cireng.2013.02.018.

12. Brewer JO, Navaratne L, Marchington SW, Martínez Cecilia D, Quiñones Sampedro J, Muñoz Bellvis L, et al. Porcine Aortorenal artery (PARA) model for laparoscopic transcystic common bile duct exploration: the evolution of a training model to meet new clinical needs. Langenbeck's Arch Surg [Internet] 2021;2–7. Available from: https://doi.org/10.1007/s00423-020-02045-0.

13. Isla A. Laparoscopic common bile duct exploration with Mr Alberto Isla. Webinar [Internet]. London General Surgicl Skills Progam. Available from: https://zoom.us/webinar/register/WN__JuZIH9dQjKBE9iVtTYQTQ

14. Isla A. Biliary Cases Quiz with Mr Alberto Isla [Internet]. London General Surgical Skills Progam. 2020. Available from: https://zoom.us/webinar/register/WN_qnJG8hDFSlSX1wIvptlAHQ

15. Rods & Cones [Internet]. [cited 2021 Apr 9]. Available from: https://www.rods-cones.com

16. Proximie [Internet]. [cited 2021 Apr 9]. Available from: https://proximie.com

17. SPI Surgical Process Instutute [Internet]. [cited 2021 Apr 7]. Available from: https://www.sp-institute.com